Weight Loss Psychology:

How to control the behavior of weight management

Lina Psouni

First published in Greece 2013

Designed by Psouni Afroditi

Content

1. Psychology of Obesity

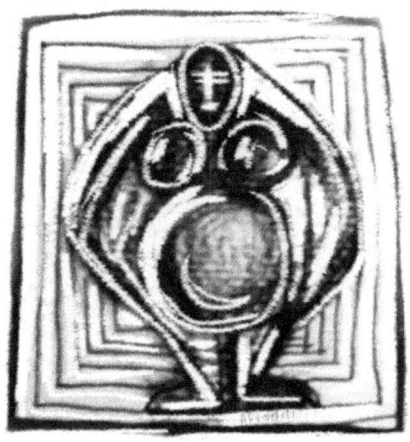

Obesity is defined as excessive accumulation of body fat. The percentage of body fat in an overweight people is higher than 18% in men and 25% in women. When the percentage of body fat is higher than 30% this person is obese.

Obese and overweight people are at an increased risk of developing health problems. Obesity has a negative impact on quality of life in a combination with health problems. Some of the health complications are presented below:

- **Diabetes** – is a metabolic disease in which blood levels of sugar are increased. There is an insulin disregulation and sugar is not controlled. It can cause many complications in the body such as cardiovascular disease, kidney failure, vision damages, nervous system apoptosis, coma etc.

- **Hypertension** – is the increase of blood pressure over normal levels. That pressure pushes the blood more than normal in arterial walls. Hypertension can cause various diseases such as atherosclerosis and vascular injury, damages to eyes and kidney.

- **Cardiovascular problems** – heart attack when an artery is blocked and cannot pump blood to the heart. Stroke when the blood supply to an area of the brain cells stops taking oxygen and be destroyed.

- **Sleeping disorders**- sleep apnea when breath is interrupted during the sleep. Snoring and poor sleep quality, and the body does not rest enough and there is fatigue during the day.

- **Veins insufficiency**- veins carry blood from all parts of the body to the heart. In cases of insufficiency veins do not function properly, there is problem of the valves and thrombosis development.

- **Osteoarthritis** – is a degenerative joint disease. Loss of cartilage and bone destruction. Result is reduced mobility, pain, atrophy of muscles and ligaments. Serious cause of osteoarthritis is obesity.

- **Menstrual cycle disorders in women-very low or very height** body weight can cause hormonal disorders in women and cause changes in menstrual cycle.

- **Some forms of cancer-** as like colon cancer, cancer of esophagus and stomach could be caused by obesity.

- **Psychological disorders** - such as low self esteem, depressive symptoms, anxiety, distorted body image etc.

WARNING: Studies have shown that someone who has normal weigh but eats junk food can possibly display more health problems than someone who is overweight but eats healthily.

Body Mass Index

Our body weight usually measured in pounds, but that number does not evaluate our body composition. A simple way to assess body composition is the Body Mass Index (BMI). BMI is a measurement that everybody could use. Is the type:

BMI= Weight (Kg)/ Height (m^2)

The values which are used most by international organizations are:

< 18,5 Kg/m^2	Underweight
18,5-25 Kg/m^2	Normal
> 25 Kg/m^2	Overweight
> 30 Kg/m^2	Obesity
> 40 Kg/m^2	Severe obesity

For example a person who is 60 kilos and 1.70 m calculates the BMI as follows. 60/1,7*1,7=20,7. According the table above this person is at normal levels. Similarly a person who is 110 kg and has height 1,70m his BMI is 110/1,7*1,7=38,06. This person as showed in the above table as obese.

BMI is an easy measurement to calculate, but sometimes it could classify people in a different category. For instance somebody who has developed his muscle mass will be heavier. That is because the muscles are heavier than fat. So the BMI of this person could be shown as overweight, but the fat of his body is in normal. For a correct calculation of the body mass, we should use fat measurement.

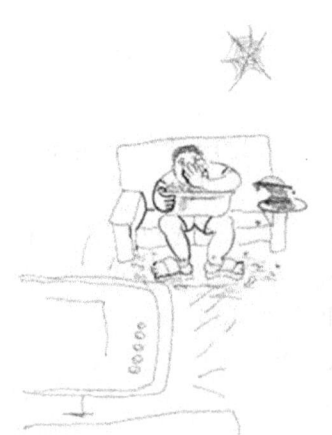

What leads us to obesity?

Inheritance is a very important factor which is responsible for the extra kilos for some people. Heredity may be associated with various diseases or hormonal disorders, such as thyroid problems. New studies suggest that there are genes which are associated with obesity.

Another factor associated with obesity is not only the environment in which we have grown but also the environment in which we live. Important role in maintaining a proper weight are having eating habits we have adopted from our family. The sedentary way of life and lack of exercise unfortunately exacerbate the problem of obesity.

The media and advertisements also contribute to increase food consumption as like the type of food which we choose. It has observed that people who watch TV consume more sweets and chocolates than those who do not see. Certainly the daily exposure to temptations influences the choices of our food.

Psychological reasons that drive us to obesity

Psychological reasons that drive us to obesity are many and different for each one, according to our experiences, our character and personality. Many of these factors coexist. Below are listed the most important:

- **Emotional relief** – the feeling of satisfaction caused by food intake, reduces intense, emotions and covers the emotional gaps. We are often leaded to overeating seeking for coverage or replacement of emotions. The result is the recruitment of more calories that we need.

- **Regression** - feelings of security that causes the food to child and infant years. During infancy we equate eating with feelings of safety and satisfaction. In adulthood, when one doesn't feel safe or secure is led to food consumption to gain those feelings which are combined with food.

- **Self-punishment** is a repeatedly behavior seen by overweight people. Usually the way of self punishment is to overeat until food causes pain in the stomach. At the same time the pain is also psychological because is accompanied by feelings of failure. The result in this case is the high calorie intake.

- **Connecting eating behaviors** with some specific situations or other behaviors, such as when we are watching TV or when we are with friends, when we are sitting on the pc, etc.

- **Negative thoughts** reduce the self-confidence, expectations and self efficacy. Negative thoughts usually make difficult the beginning of an effort difficult like a foal achievement. Negative thoughts are common in overweight people and usually involve feeling of failure not only for the body weight but also in other parts of their life.

- **Self fulfilling prophecy** is to behave according to the characteristics that our environment has attributed to us. For example the overweight child receives messages from his family and from his environment which define the profile of an overweight person. This child learns to behave adopting these features. Also, the child believes that it will never manage to lose his weight. The same thing is happening with adults. Many obese or overweight adults believe that they will never be able to slim down. This idea prevents them from doing any effective effort to lose weight.

- **Dependence/addiction** has been found that occurs with some foods with high levels of fat, high levels of sugar and salt. Those examples are fast foods, chocolates, sweets etc.

- **Being rejected** creates intense gaps which people seek to cover by food intake. Rejection could be in sexual life, in business, in social life etc.

- **Movement of the source** of the problems to other causes. In these cases psychological problems are replaced with obesity. For example if somebody suffers from anxiety it could appears as a disordered body image. The same could be happen to someone who is depressed and shows problems associated with high body weight.

- **Denial of the source** of the problem. Other times we deny the source of a problem and blame external causes or people. In these cases, the problem is appeared differently. Obesity replaces anxiety problems. For example somebody who is overweight considers they have a disorder body image and does not show the usual symptoms of anxiety. The same could be happen with someone who is depressed and shows the problems associated with his weight.

- **Hiding or disappearing the source** of the problem. The denial of the source of the problem is another way of hiding or disappearing. ". For example someone who is overweight attaches the liability of his obesity to the environment and denies that he has a problem.

- **The denial of reality** happens when we try to hide in our subconscious the truth, knowledge, experiences memories or feelings. Many times obese people do not accept the situation, the size of the problem and also the amount of food that they eat. In most cases obese people avoid thinking and analyze the situation of their weight.

- Other times a **reaction** appeared in our behavior. The reaction is often the opposite than the one desired. This is the reason why we respond in a negative way to diets. Also, the theory of reactance describes those opposite reactions.

- **Incomplete sexual life** could cause frustration, depression and severe stress. The decreased sexual satisfaction is often substituted by overeating. Some foods like chocolate are related with the replacement of sexual impulses.

The vicious cycle of obesity

When these behaviors are repeated, they become habits which result negatively in weight gain. Behaviors cause weight increase and weight increase cases specific behaviors. This is the vicious cycle of obesity. Increased body weight lowers our self-esteem and self-confidence and causes negative feelings. People who are frustrated by their appearance create self-destructive behaviors and end up with overeating.

The following figure shows the vicious cycle of obesity. It seems that our behavior causes an increase in food intake, which in turn, causes again the same behavior.

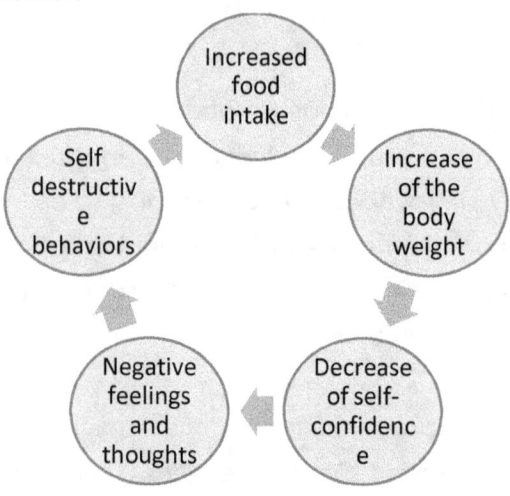

Let's ask ourselves:
- *According to the above what is happening to myself?*
- *What affects my behavior?*
- *What am I trying to replace or cover by food intake?*
- *Which is my vicious cycle?*

Psychological profile of overweight people

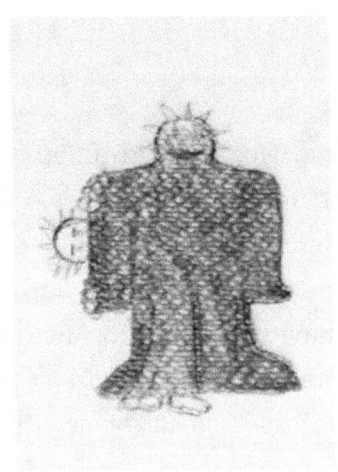

Someone with extra pounds almost has low self-confidence as like low self-esteem. That person underestimates himself and feels that he will not be successful in anything. Simultaneously he is not happy with his looks because of his body image. Repeated failures in getting slim efforts and unfulfilled goals reduce the already low self confidence.

Frustration of our self brings negative thoughts and negative emotions. The combination of these two is the worst that someone can do to an already negative psychology. The bad psychological situation usually accompanied by destructive thoughts results in a low motivation towards achieving losing weight.

In addition overweight people have a low self-control. The low self control is negatively reinforced by low confidence, negative thoughts and negative emotions. So the self-control as a behavior does not have many changes to be improved. On the contrary, it results in disappointment and dissatisfaction for the lack of self-control.

The overweight person often hides unconsciously behind the extra pounds. Avoiding their sexual life or competition may be some of that reasons why the connection of the person with the bulky body image may satisfy unscrupulous goals and give a sense of security. Sometimes, an overweight person cannot accept his new image and cannot redefine his role if he loses weight. This is also a serious factor that blocks slimming achievement.

Stigmatization of overweight people

In western societies obesity is highly criticized. Negative attitudes are developed, which in turn are lead to negative behaviors towards overweight people. Studies have shown that negative attitudes about overweight people are identified even in 3 years old children. Like adults, overweight children are victims of social stigmatization. Unfortunately children have a negative attitude against obese people and also against themselves. All these negative stereotypes can have significant negative effects on social development during childhood and puberty.

All the above does not mean that every overweight
or obese people has psychological problems.
Psychological analysis and support could be very
effective to lose weight

Adults are often treated with prejudice because of their weight. For example it has been observed that health professionals have negative attitudes about overweight people. It has also been observed that women are more stigmatized than men. Generally, overweight people are attributed as lazy, gluttonous, with a lack of confidence, unable, whit a lack of self control etc. All these factors lead overweight people to blame their selves and this is the worst thing that somebody could do to himself.

Overweight people who lose weight shows:

→ Improvement in their psychology

→ Improvement in their mood

→ Decrease in depressive symptoms

→ Improvement in social interactions

→ Improvement in self-confidence

2. Body image

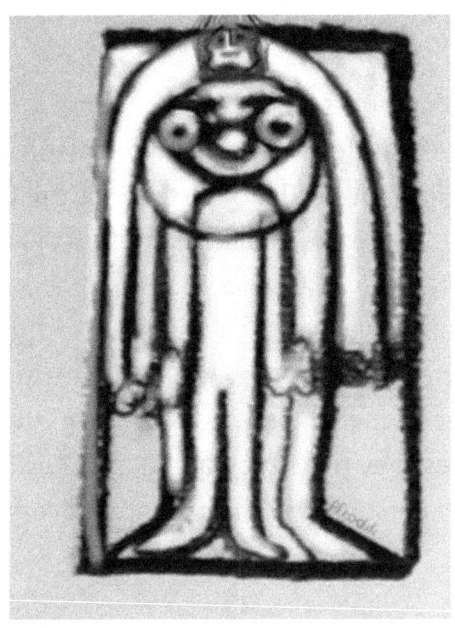

Body image as a psychological term is what impression each person has for the appearance of the body. Body image is not how we really look like. It is certain that our personality and behavior is affected by our body image. The wrong impression we may have for ourselves may be the main reason for a psychological disorder. For example, people suffering from anorexia nervosa tent to think they are overweight but in real life they are very slim. So, there is a disturbed perception of the real fact.

The acceptance or the non acceptance of our body image from the society is the reason why all those problems are caused. Our appearance plays an important role in the progress of our life. For example, it has been noticed that good looking people are more likely to find a job. Also, at court cases good looking people are rarely judged guilty.

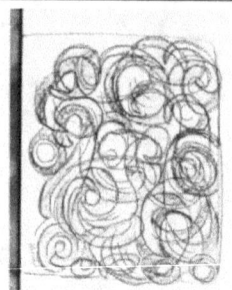

The acceptance from our society owing to body image accompanies people throughout their life. Surely many people, if not everyone, have seen or remember from our childhood some fat children to be picked on at school and being ignored by their classmates. Unlike the good looking ones who are usually popular at school.
Even attractive people stare at their reflexion in the mirror because of insecurity and not because of vanity. Studies have shown that attractive people haven't got a higher self esteem than the average number. Whereas many times they think they are judged for their beauty ignoring their behavior and personality which is something that reduces their whole self-esteem.

In general, women are judged much more on their appearance than men. They receive the pressure to keep their appearance according to the (role) models of modern age. Studies have shown that when awe look at pictures of very skinny models we may feel sad, stress, guilt, embarrassment and insecurity about our appearance. Eight out of ten women are not satisfied with their appearance. We can feel disappointment about our body appearance when our mood is bad, which shows that our body is connected to our attitude. Also we feel disappointment about our body when we have been picked on because of our appearance since we were kids, when we did not exercise and after a large consumption of food.

Our body image is associated with:

- Self confidence
- Self esteem
- Mood disorders
- Behavioral disorders
- Stress
- Anger towards our self and the society
- Self criticism

Body image development

In ancient times the ideal body for men was the natural muscled body while women seemed to have curves and extra pounds. In 1500 the female body was bell shaped with a large periphery and small breasts. Women wore corsets pushing their breasts to look smaller. In 1700 corsets were so tied creating several health problems. In 1800-1900 the perfect body was plump, with tiny waist and gave emphasis to the hips and buttocks

In early 1900 most lean women became fashionable. Women began to be interested in sport and ideal weight. From 1920 women with very small breasts were fashionable. Also in the early 1900 was born the plastic surgery of the face. In 1918 the book "diet and health" became a bestseller.

In the '30s brought back corset in combination with lean hips. In the '50s Marilyn Monroe brings back in fashion the curvy body. In the'60 lean body became the most important indicator of physical attractiveness when Twiggy appeared. She weighs just 40 pounds and her height was 1,70m. Also, the Barbie doll appeared that period with the unnatural body.

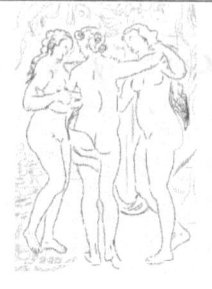

In 1970 hippies were in fashion but women still liked to have impossibly thin waist and large breasts. In 1975 the top models weighed 8% less than the average woman. After 1980 lean body remained an ideal body but it was required to be also toned but curvy. The fashion then was dieting and exercising. In the early '90s lean body became more fashionable and increased the interest of women in sports. Pamela Anderson had the ideal body. Today's models weigh 23% less than the average woman, while are using many artificial means to achieve a better body image.

Influences on body image

Media and body image

The psychological pressure for the best body image is becoming more intense by the daily unlimited advertising of the media. Constantly are displayed messages about beauty which are perceived consciously or unconsciously and define our beauty standards.

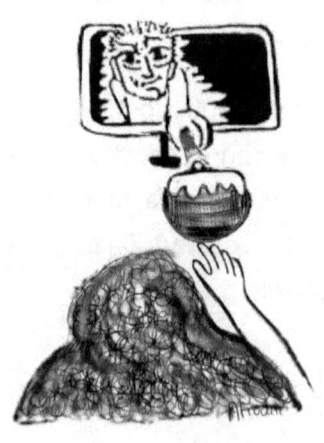

All this deluge of information about body image leads us to the constant search for improvement. That improvement helps people to accept their body and reduces body image disorders. Unfortunately, if people aren't satisfied by their looks and if there is no improvement, the results are the exact.

Children's toys

The dolls for little girls are a serious cause that could lead to excessive diets.

The dolls' bodies look very beautiful and no one realizes that it is abnormal. If the Barbie doll was a normal woman she would be about 54 kg and 1,82m in height. Compared to the average, a normal woman is about 66 kg and 1,65m in height. Also the average woman would have to make the following unrealistic changes to become as the doll:

- to increase the breast periphery by 13 cm
- to raise the neck by 7,5 cm
- to reduce by 15 cm her waist periphery

No little girl when playing with dolls does not think all the above. The most common thought is to compare their body with the doll's and how they will achieve this body. Children should have some knowledge to criticize and judge these toys so that toys would not affect them.

In the contrary, the boys' toys provide the muscular "huge" body. The ideal man of our days is muscular, with a shortage of fat and hairless. The ideal body has the shape of V with broad shoulders and skinny torso and legs. Unfortunately, the average man has very little chance to achieve it without having to:

- be developed extreme and unnatural
- use extreme exercise
- do extreme diets
- Make use of supplement and anabolic substances

Let's ask ourselves ...
We see pictures of toys providing imaginary
or supernatural body image.

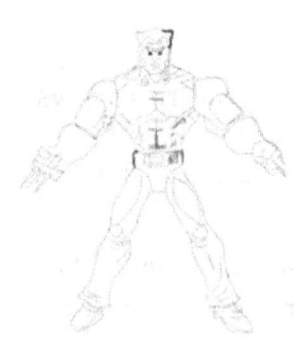

- *How can these images affect the children?*
- *Can I remember what it was affected me when I was a kid?*

Advertisements

Most of the times, advertisements show pictures of beautiful bodies and beautiful people as models for the ideal life. If we look carefully almost all the advertisements provide thin women and muscled men. Also, advertisements correlate the image of a beautiful toned body in men and the image of a thin woman with a successful life.

Extreme processing of photos and video are made so well that it is difficult to be recognized. Rarely do we take into account the entire computer processing in perfect bodies and faces which are well hidden behind the messages of the ads. Sometimes the result of that processing is too unnatural and makes us realize it. A good advice is that when we watch TV or when we read magazines we should recognize all the fake ideal lives and not let ourselves to make unconscious comparisons which are leading to disappointments.

Exercise:

We see the pictures in magazines, on the internet, on TV, people who have the perfect body...

- *How does the ideal body affect our standards?*
- *How much does it affect us?*
- *Could we remember of an ad that displays a nice body? Lets assess that add by answering the following questions:*
  - *How is shown the ideal body?*
  - *Are the people in the advertisements being found in real life?*
  - *What are the messages that advertisements give?*
  - *Is there any element of the product that is not referred?*
  - *Are there lies?*
  - *Are there excessive elements?*
  - *Are they using someone famous to pass on their messages?*
- *To what extent do I criticize myself for my appearance?*
- *How much do I judge others based on their appearance?*

2.Psychology of diet

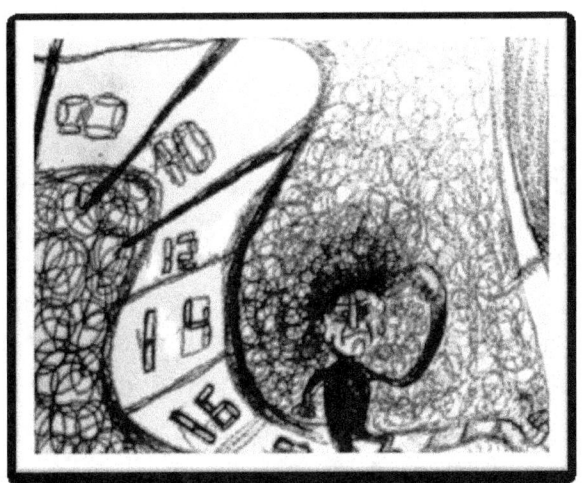

Diet for our body

We diet when we reduce the calories we consume to burn calories for weight loss. The strict diets that are suggested for fast weight loss are good neither for our health nor our psychology. It is shown below how dangerous diets are for our bodies. Most people have very high expectations to lose too much pounds in a short period of time. The huge and sudden reduction of food can cause various problems to our body because we do not take all the nutrients that are necessary.

Wrong diets can cause health problems such as:

- Fatigue
- Dizziness
- Dehydration
- Hair Loss
- Osteoporosis
- Dry Skin
- Inability to concentrate
- Disturbances in women's menstrual circle
- Headache

A research done on animals showed increased levels of anxiety like symptoms of depresive behavior. It was imprortant that some genes that regulate stress and diet were altered. As a result of the diet the animals eat much more than before in stress conditions. After the diet period the animals return to their normal diet and weight but their changes in stress behaviors to the food remained in their DNA.

CAUTION: Sliming drugs that are sold commercially and promise easy slimming have very serious side effects. Some of these drugs are not approved and are illegal. Also some need a prescription but people try them without doctor' advise. Some of the side effects from sliming drugs are:

- mood changes
- blood pressure increase
-fast pulse rate
-palpitations

- heart problems
-insomnia
-constipation
-sweating
-headache

Stress and anxiety on a diet

Diets cause stress and anxiety. We suffer stress when we force ourselves for some reason and anxiety when we afraid for failure. Stress and anxiety are two major reasons that we might discontinue the diet.

Stress while being on a diet is caused by the pressure to ourselves when we reduce the amount of food. If we feel restricted in our dietary choices, or if we feel committed to the slimming program then probably we suffer from stress. A diet under stress condition is very difficult to be achieved.

We feel anxiety while dieting when we are afraid that we will be hungry all the time and we will lose the pleasure of our food. In addition, we cause anxiety symptoms when we believe that the diet will be unsuccessful. In conclusion the diet is causing stress with limited amount of food and anxiety because of the expected results. This combination guarantees the failure!

Self confidence and self esteem

Self-confidence is the belief in ourselves that we are able to achieve the goals that we set. Somebody who has a high self-confidence believes in himself and somebody who has low confidence believes that he will fail. High self-confidence is an important factor for a successful effort of weight loss. The failed attempts for slimming or have lost weight and regained pounds but on diets are negative factors for self-confidence. Someone who has repeatedly failed to lose weight, it doesn't believe in his power when he starts a new diet.

Self esteem is the impression that we have for ourselves. Self-esteem is high when we are satisfied with ourselves and decreased when we are disappointed. The failed attempts for slimming and frustration from the image of our body reduce our overall self-esteem. High self esteem associated with high confidence and contributes significantly to the success of weight loss.

Self punishment and self destruction

Self punishment and self destruction are ways to relief ourselves of our emotions. Usually, when we are disappointed of ourselves unconsciously or consciously we want to punish ourselves.

The feelings of anger towards ourselves could easily lead us to the destruction. Generally, anger feelings should be defused or be controled. If that feelings are connected with the weight loss program, we will have the opposite effect than the expected.

Also feelings of depression could lead us to self-destruction. Freud's theory relates self-destruction with the instinct of death and claims that we lead ourselves to death during ourlife.

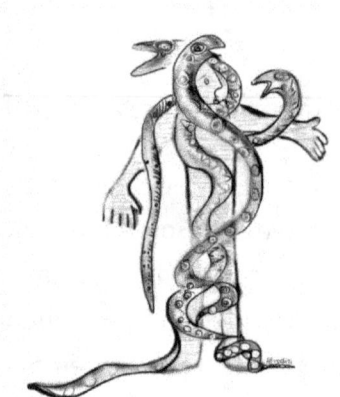

Reactance theory

Reactance theory is a reactive behavior to the prohibited things or to the elimination of freedoms. When a desired behavior is banned, the person feels that the freedom is challenged and tries to claim it in every way.

With this in mind, that person evaluates more positively the forbidden behavior. For example, in a diet program there are many forbidden foods. If the person feels restricted he could easily express a different and opposite behavior than the proposed. This theory explains various outbursts and irregularities during the diet program. At the same time an aggressive behavior could be developed towards ourselves and towards others who come in on diet.

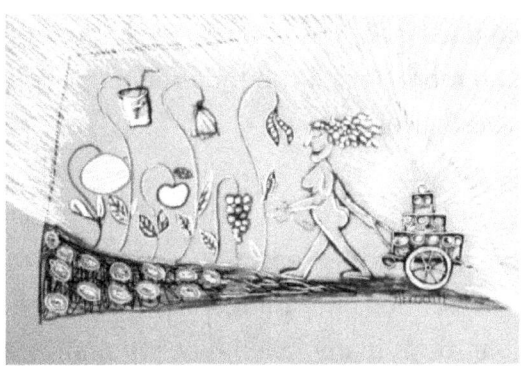

The mistakes in diets

The biggest mistake that people make in diet is setting a very high goal. Also they have high expectations of themselves in a very little period of time. A goal to lose too many pounds seems unrealistic to everybody. In addition a high goal could cause stress and anxiety. It is much better if we set a goal to change of the way of living than the weight loss. For sure if we achieve to change our way of life we will also achieve to control our weight.

Another huge mistake is the impression that we will be on a diet for a specific period of time and then return to our old habits. The "miracle diet" unfortunately does not exist. We come again to the conclusion that a permanent change of lifestyle will lead to permanent results in weight control.

As mentioned above a serious mistake in diets is the large calorie reduction. If we reduce dramatically the calories intake, our body will be under stress conditions and it is completely normal our body to react. That way larger and more abrupt the food reduction is, the more chances of fail and quit the diet program.

The body has the tendency to try to return to the balance that was used to his previous weight. For this reason when we skip meals or when we reduce the amount of food, the hunger symptoms become even more pronounced. In long term many failed diet attempts lead to weight gain rather than loss.

A psychological mistake in the diets is the connection of food intake with pleasure. People who diet set rules to themselves and they feel that they lose the pleasures in life. If we feel deprivation in a diet program, we are bound to fail. The diet should give us a positive feedback and be a behavior that we enjoy doing.

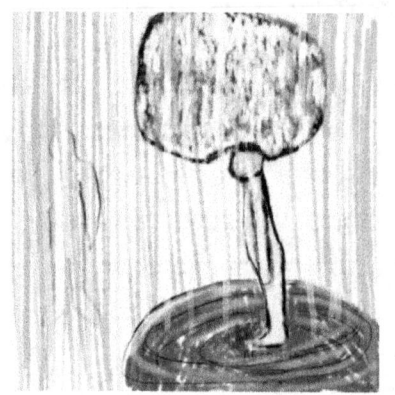

The vicious cycle through dieting

If the results of pressing diets are negative, we could be driven to feelings of frustration, anger and self-destruction. That easily creates the vicious cycle of failed diet. Someone who is stressed when doing a diet it is 100% sure that he'll fail. That failure will cause intense negative emotional feelings and self-destruction. The increasing of food is the next step to relieve those feelings. The final result will be the increased body weight and negative feelings.

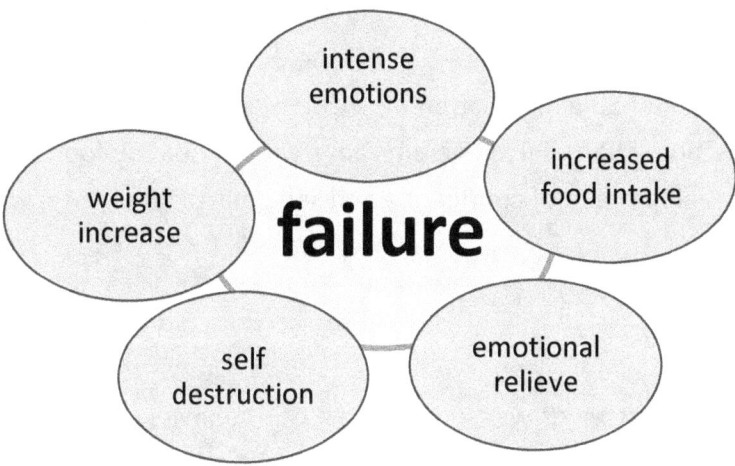

Let's think about...

- *Does it happen to me when I try to control myself?*
- *How many times have I made an effort to get slim?*
- *Why did I abandon the effort each time?*
- *Why I thinking that the diet program didn't work on me?*

To achieve diet

The first goal to lose weight should be the personal balance instead of the battle with the scales. Anyone who starts to lose weight should first of all be determined to:

- Change his life
- Be relaxed

The only certain way to achieve weight loss is a changing our lifestyle. We have to apply the following behaviors to get results and lose weight:

→ Application of daily exercise
→ The understanding of satiation
→ The disconnection of positive emotions with unhealthy foods
→ The developments of confidence and self control

Self awareness

Going deeper into ourselves we try to explain our behavior. That analysis could be assisted by answering the following questions:

- *When did the failed diets problem start?*
- *What caused the diets to fail?*
- *Why can't achieve my diet goals?*
- *What were my eating habits in the past?*
- *What has happened now to start a new behavior?*
- *What are the consequences?*

Self-observation

Observation of ourselves before, during and after, any behavior will lead us to valuable conclusions. Sometimes we do not realize the emotional background of a behavior like the thoughts that accompany behaviors or emotions. When we are aware of our feelings and the caused-connected behaviors we can control them more easily. If we frequently repeat some eating habits then we connect eating with some behaviors and then we seek to repeat them continuously.

For example, common behaviors are eating while we are watching TV, when we are using the pc, or when we are with friends. Most of the time eating includes unhealthy foods such as chips, crisps, popcorn and soft drinks. We will see afterwards how we can use the technique of self observation.

Let's observe...

- *Before we consume any food if we are really hungry or if we are looking to eat something out of habit.*
- *After the consumption of a food we observe if we are full up.*
- *If any emotion leads us to food consumption (e.g. Anxiety, depression, anger, joy, etc.)*
- *We observe the feeling that is caused by intake of a particular type of food.*

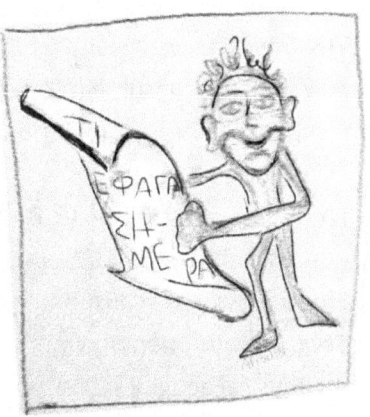

Table to record habits

In the following table we record everyday eating habits. We record the time of consumption, the amount of food, the feelings, the place and if we were alone or accompanied by somebody. Also we should ask ourselves before our food intake if we were hungry and after if the food was enough. All that details will show us if we associate food intake with specific behaviors, specific emotions or if we eat because we connect eating with socializing.

Time	Amount of food	Hunger/fill out	Emotion	Place	People

Ideal is to record the following habits (for a week or 3 days at least):
- The time
- Any food we consume (food or drink)
- Hunger scale from 1 to 5 (hunger: 1=not at all, 5=very much)
- Fill in scale after food consumption   (full up: 1=not at all, 5=very much)
- Emotional consumption (If a feeling led us to food, e.g. Anger anxiety, depression)
- Emotion which is caused from food intake
- Total consumption of water
- All Physical activity

4. Emotions

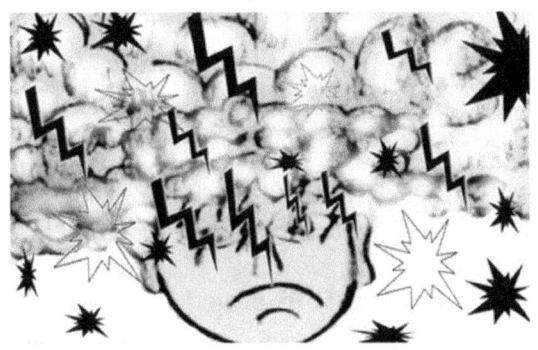

Emotions are psycho-physiological responses of the human to the environment. Emotions are causing biological changes to prepare the body to the external conditions. Emotions affect our thoughts and our behavior. The intensity of the emotions based to the size of the stimulus and the frequency of occurrence. For example fear prepares the body to face any threat. The nervous system is stimulated and ready for "fight or flight".

Physiology of emotions

Physiology of emotions shows how emotions are created, how they affect our body and which are physical symptoms that they are caused by them.

Neurotransmitters

Neurotransmitters are the chemicals are acting in our brain and regulate our emotions. Neurotransmitters are used to transfer information from one neuron of our brain to another. The most important neurotransmitters are the following:

- Dopamine-regulates alertness, energy, depression
- Norepinephrine- regulates attention, pleasure, reward
- Serotonin- regulates mood, calmness, relaxation

Individuals who have emotional disorders have increased or decreased levels of neurotransmitters. It has been proven that when somebody has overcome an emotional disorder the levels of neurotransmitters return to normal levels. This could be done either by medication or psychotherapy. If we know that our emotions are the result of the level and the movement of neurotransmitters, we could understand how our brain works.

In turn, neurotransmitters are influenced by substances as like alcohol, tobacco, drugs, caffeine and even some foods. Also neurotransmitters are affected by diseases such as diabetes, heart diseases, allergies, hormonal disorders etc. Also they could be affected from our way of life, lack of sleep and exercise. It has been found that people who do not sleep the required hours can put on weight. It is also known that exercise increases endorphins associated with enjoyment and pleasure.

Foods that affect our mood

- **Carbohydrate** - helps release serotonin to increase energy and alertness.

- **Protein** – contains amino acids tyrosine and helps to release dopamine and epinephrine, which reduces stress, increases calmness, better sleep and reduce appetite.

- **Sugar** – increases insulin release, increase energy but for a short while.

- **Dairy products** - contain tryptophan which helps to release the serotonin, calm the nerves and induce a better sleep.

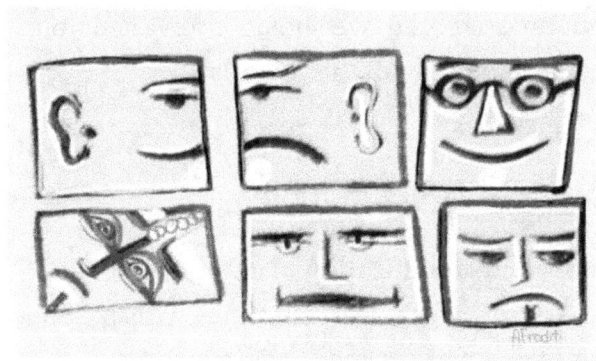

Control of emotions

To test our feelings we should be able to recognize the emotional condition of ourselves, as like the emotions of people who are around us. It is also important the recognition of the influence of emotions in our behavior. People who have a high emotional intelligence also have in control of their emotions, regardless of external conditions.

Emotional intelligence includes the understanding of self, objectives, intentions and related behavior. In addition, it includes the understanding of others, their behavior and emotions.

It has been demonstrated that emotional intelligence can be developed and practiced

On the whole, the most important step for emotion control is to understand them. The recognition of emotions but also understanding why they are caused will help us to predict their appearance. If we understand that prediction we can prevent it. That could happen when we feel that an emotion is created, we should intervene in our thoughts and do not allow the development of that emotion.

Strategies to control our emotions

1. Self-awareness and identification of emotions

We must be able to recognize the emotions which influence our behaviors. Those emotions are changed over time. Also, we should be able to recognize the emotions of other people from their reactions and their behaviors, as like their body language. Many behaviors are explained if we understand the emotions that cause them.

2. Awareness in daily basis

Secondly, we have to develop the individual awareness of emotions on a daily basis. We have to observe how our emotions affect the way that we react to new situations. In addition we must be able to evaluate the intensity of our emotions.

3. Separation of thoughts and feelings

We must understand how our emotions can influence our thoughts. For example we can observe that when we are angry we are thinking about things that are vindictive about others and when the anger passes we think in a completely different way.

4. Determination of the strategies to control emotions

We can develop our own strategies for regulating our emotions. For example positive thinking, positive self-talk, even listening more music, exercising etc could be helpful to control our feelings.

5. Goal settings for emotional management

When we understand our emotions the next step is to control them by setting the correct goals. For example, the avoidance of negative behaviors of anger could be a goal for somebody with anger problems.

6. The applications of positive self talk

The development of an appropriate self talk could be very helpful to control our thoughts which influence our emotions. The change of our emotions cannot happen directly but indirectly if we can control our self talk and our thoughts.

7. Role playing (real or imagery)

Role playing is a very effective method to work with our emotions. Role playing games are also more effective when are recorded.

For the better results in managing emotions the person should:
→ Have self control
→ Remain optimistic
→ Express the emotions
→ Trying to understand the emotions of others
→ Develop the ability to understand body language

→ Be flexible in the way that explains behaviors

→ To follow his emotions rather than banish them

When we know and understand our feelings and our behaviors then we are able to control them.

Function of emotions

The following image presents how the emotions interact with the physical symptoms and thoughts. In other words how the external stimulus can cause emotions, thoughts and physical symptoms. In the example of the image the stimulus is an ice cream which creates the following:

- Body responses, for example salivation
- Emotional arousal, for example pleasure, delight, tranquility
- Thoughts, positive or negative

All these effects aroused by the sight of one ice cream. They are developed according to our experiences in our lives. The most important is to understand that physical symptoms, emotions and thoughts are interrelated, have developed together and one brings the other.

For example, the thought of one ice cream could cause a physical stimulation and the corresponding emotions. The same happens in the existence of an emotion. That emotion can cause a thought and the thought can cause the physical response. This is a common chain reaction when we seek a particular food to alleviate our emotions.

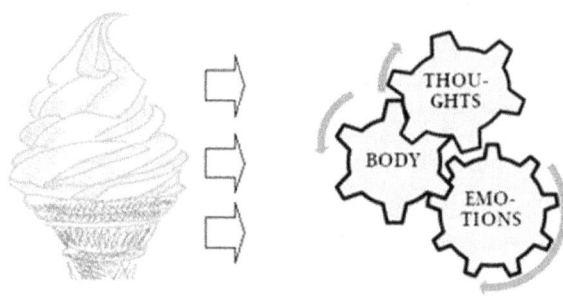

Emotions and food intake

Many behaviors occur and depend on our emotional state. Associating emotions with specific behaviors becomes a habit when it is repeated many times. Some of these behaviors are related to food intake. Many times we connect emotional relief with the consumption of specific foods.

By observing our behavior and correlating it with our emotional state we can collect a lot of information about our eating habits. The following symptoms lead us to a huge consumption of food.

Stress	Fear
Depression	Panic
Anxiety	Apathy
Boredom	Guilt
Shame	Remorse

Let' think...
- *How do I connect my emotions with food intake?*
- *What are my thoughts before I eat?*
- *How important is food to me?*

- *Do I relieve my emotions with food?*
- *How do I feel after eating?*
- *Why can't I control myself?*

Emotional hunger

Emotional hunger is the connection of our emotional state with food intake. Emotional hunger is not a real need to our bodies. It is the need of relieving our emotions by eating. That relieve becomes a habit during our life time.

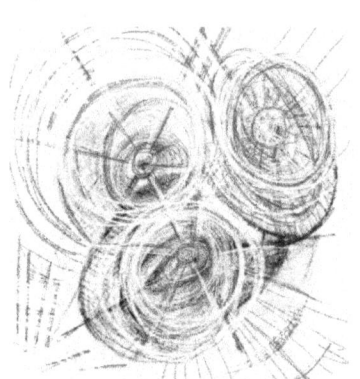

Emotional hunger is an acquired and not a real need. For example, if we give chocolate to a small child who cries, we learn to relieve the feelings of sorrow with sweet food. So he learns to seek for specific foods when he has specific feelings. The same could happen if we connect a category of foods with emotions according to our experience. Below the differences between real hunger and emotional hunger are presented.

Emotional hunger	Real hunger
o Comes suddenly o Is related to certain foods o Only certain foods will satisfy us o We seek instant gratification o After food intake we feel guilty	o Comes gradually o Most of foods will meet our need o Withstand a few more minutes before eating something o After lunch we have the sense of satisfaction

Respectively we connect food intake with pleasure. Feasts and celebrations have been associated with excessive food intake. We also believe that in order to enjoy it, we have to eat as much as we can.

- *How would we feel if we held a feast or a party with only with healthy foods?*
- *Would it be accepted by our environment?*
- *Would it be negatively criticized?*

The foods which are associated with relief or cause some emotions are called pleasure foods. Essentially all people connect to foods and feelings during their lifetime. The environment that we grow up is very crucial in the creation of those connections.

It has been observed that when we are happy we usually consume foods like pizza and steaks. When we are depressed we prefer something sweet, like chocolates and ice creams. When we are bored we choose snacks such as crisps, nuts and foods that require repetitive movements.

Emotional control and food consumption

We see the first step to control our emotions is to recognize them. The same happens to the behaviors which are associated with emotions. We should learn to recognize emotional hunger and distinguish it from the real hunger. To do that, we observe the specific conditions and the specific thoughts which drive us to emotional hunger. Usually these thoughts and emotions are similar and are repeated very often.

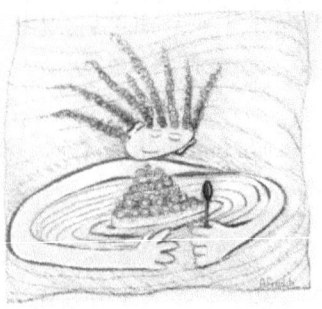

At the same time, we can observe which are the foods that we prefer according to our emotional state. Generally which is the kind of food that we seek? For example is something salty or sweet? Is it a type of a food with a high percentage of a fat and a rich flavor? Is it something absolutely specific?

We have taken the first step, when we know that our hunger is emotional and not real. If we keep a diet plan with no big gaps between meals, we also know that the hunger we feel is not real. The realization of the kind of hunger is very crucial for a successful slimming. If we frequently repeat some eating habits, then we learn to apply them every day. For example, a common behavior is eating while watching TV. Most of the time eating includes junk foods. We could help ourselves to quit the emotional hunger in theory and in practice, by following the tips:

- We should avoid buying the specific foods that we desire when we are emotional concerned. If we have not those foods in the house we could prevent outbursts and uncontrolled consumption.
- We change our behavior in order to satisfy our emotions differently. Exercising for example is the perfect way to relief our emotions.
- We try to replace unhealthy food with other lighter and healthier. We do not need to push ourselves we can consume something different and lighter.
- We try to moderate food consumption and not deprive ourselves. It is better to eat a small chocolate than to leave it for a long time. In the end the amount of chocolate will be much bigger because of our desire.
- We recognize the sense of satisfaction and know that we should stop after taking a reasonable amount of food.

- *According to these data, what drives us to food consumption?*

Emotional control and exercise

Like emotions and diet something similar happens in emotions and exercise. The attitude towards exercising is very important. That is how we consider the benefits from exercise, like thinking how difficult or easy it is to perform. Some people consider exercising healthy while others believe they are forced to do it. Who is more likely to exercise regularly?

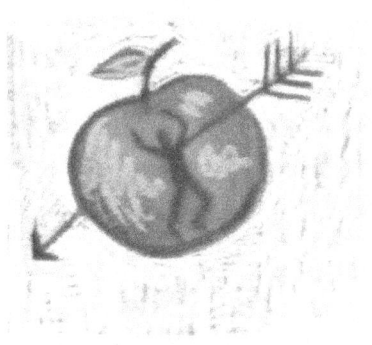

- *Which are the emotions we associate exercise with? We avoid exercising regularly or do we daily seek to do something?*

In order to have a successful fitness program, we should keep the positive feelings and eliminate the negative ones. For example a positive feeling is the reward for the daily effort. A negative feeling is the fatigue or weakness after exercise. It depends on us in which of the two we will take for ourselves. We observe to ourselves what thoughts we use before, during and after the workout. In this way we try to recognize the emotional feedback we are giving to ourselves. If we do not receive satisfaction from the exercise then we need to change our thoughts. Instead the possibilities to qult exercising are very high.

Always the rewards of exercise should be greater than the feeling of fatigue. If it is not we have to change our behavior to satisfy our feelings. If we observe that we do not reward ourselves enough then we should change it consciously. Often overweight people are very strict with themselves. They do not reward themselves if they do not see significant changes. This is a big mistake. Each small step we make we must reward ourselves to continue the behavior.

In addition, we must find forms of exercise that we prefer. Some forms of exercises are preferred according to our personality. It is better to have a variety in the types of exercises, in order to fight against boredom.

Who plays with our emotions?

Many times, advertising companies are based in the production or the relief of emotions with foods to promote a product. Their goal is to create an association of an emotion with the food that they provide. A very successful advertisement will make the product to become a need, whenever we want to cause or to relieve an emotion.

The best and more effective ads are those that display little information but include a severe emotional content. The results of advertisements with emotional content showed more positive changes in attitudes towards the product than the advertisements which use cognitive information. Even the intense negative emotion used by advertisers has been found to increase the attention to the product. Advertisers use successfully all the emotions like humor, love, enthusiasm, shame, disgust, fear and pity.

In the following pictures are shown some typical advertisements which use the methods of emotions with food.

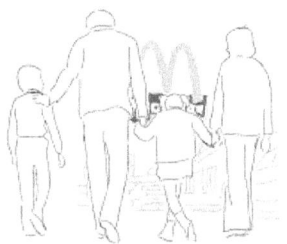

Nowadays the image of a happy family who eats in fast food restaurants is very common. It successfully connects the junk food with moments of happiness, love and family warmth.

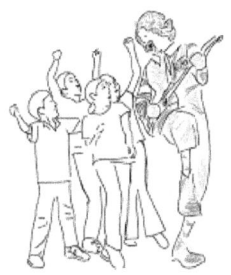

The happiness and fun of children is due to the fast food restaurants that they are visited and of course the junk food that gave them so much pleasure as shown in the picture.

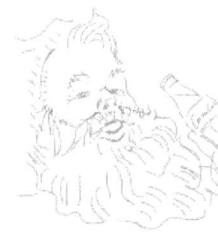

The famous picture of Santa Claus is the product of an advertising campaign for a known product. Unconsciously we associate this image with moments of happiness and family warmth. The same happens when we consume the product.

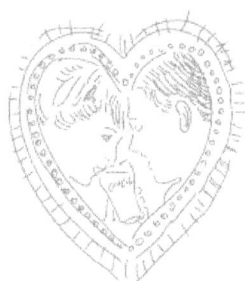

This ad is trying to recall strong feelings of love. If that connection of this is strong the consumption of the product will be increased.

5. Thoughts

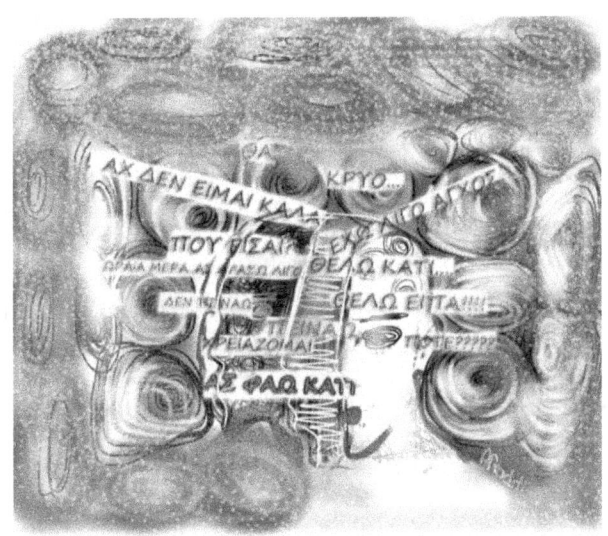

Thoughts are interdependent with the emotions and the conditions of our body. A thought could cause some feelings but also the other way round, emotions could cause thoughts. If this is repeated many times, then thoughts "jump out" without control. A stimulus is enough to cause an emotion. In turn it will cause some thoughts and in this case we have a vicious cycle which the more it is repeated, the stronger it becomes.

Anxiety is the fear of the unknown. Usually anxiety will cause thoughts of destruction. Those thoughts will increase the levels of stress, which would cause physical symptoms such as tremor and tachycardia. A stimulus that could cause anxiety is the diet program. In this way, we almost fail to follow a diet program.

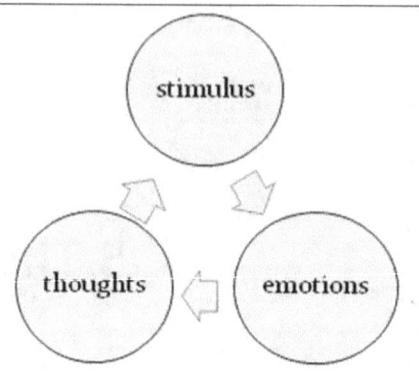

Respectively, the physical symptoms can cause thoughts, which in turn can cause some emotions. This happens in panic attack. Usually, in these cases we have a physical symptom, such as tachycardia, dizziness, trembling etc. The symptom begins with a scenario of destruction and health risk. That scenario will cause severe anxiety symptoms that will enhance the physical symptoms. Also in this case we have a vicious circle.

We should realize that changing our thinking is possible as physiology is concerned. It is possible to achieve that if we want.

The brain

Essentially thoughts are nothing more than electrical and chemical signals that make the brain cells communicate. The structures of the brain cause stimulus which are activated by neurotransmitters. The daily behaviors and thoughts change the structure and function of biochemical factors in the brain.

The connections between neurons in the brain are called synapses. These synapses constantly change. It has been found that 70% of the synapses in our brain change every day. We have 100 billion neurons in our brain; each one of which makes 10.000 new connections each second. We lose about 1.000 neurons every day, but that is compensated by the activation of others neurons and the increase of synapses. This ability is called brain plasticity.

How we can control our thoughts

We try to recognize the connection between emotions, body reactions and thoughts:

1. Observe which are our negative thoughts
2. Observe what is the connection between thoughts and feelings
3. Observe and recognize our body reactions (such as, tachycardia, tremors, increased respiration rate, sweating, stomach pain, fatigue).
4. Observe psychological symptoms (such as restlessness, inability to concentrate, confusion, negative thoughts, insomnia, decreased pleasure).
5. Observe changes in our behavior (such as rapid speech, nail biting, rapid leg movements, muscle twitching, aggression, isolation).
6. We realize that thoughts affect our body and our body reactions affect our thoughts.
7. We try to intervene in our thoughts before their creation.
8. We try to replace negative thoughts with positive thoughts.
9. We change the environment to block the connections which are related to negative thoughts.
10. We aim at the expression of our emotions rather than their accumulation.

All the above can be done as long as we want to do it. In the same way we analyze the thoughts and emotions which are associated with food intake.

1st Exercise:

The following stimulus...

- *Which emotions it causes?*
- *What are the thoughts on the subject?*
- *Where those thoughts lead me?*
- *Did the first emotion change with the thoughts?*
- *Were the thoughts changed?*
- *How do all the above affect food intake?*

Positive thoughts	Negative thoughts
• I have positive attitude about the stimulus	• I have a negative attitude for the stimulus
• It makes me happy	• It make me happy but for a while
• I keep this feeling	• Automatically I restrict it to my self
• And I increase it	• I try in moderation
• I don't forbid anything to myself	• But I don't reward myself
• I avoid negative emotions	• I consume a large amount of food
• I eat in moderation	• I feel guilty
• I reward myself for self control	• I consume the whole quantity
• I add the feeling of satisfaction	
• I distract myself by doing something else but I keep on rewarding myself	

2nd exercise:

In the diary of good intake we add the observation of our thoughts. We observe the thoughts that cause or are caused by the emotion which are associated with the consumption of food.

To change our thoughts

As we saw, first of all if we want to change our thoughts we should observe them. Then we look for the reasons causing the thoughts. The thoughts could be caused from emotions or external stimuli. Usually we react in the same way to external stimulus. We teach ourselves to think in a certain way. It is easier to change the negative thoughts before they are created. The thoughts after being created coexist with the emotions and it is a more difficult situation to change.

To help ourselves change the thoughts we could intervene in the environment. For example if we feel sad and we seeking food to relieve our pain instead we can go for a walk. If we repeat that behavior several times we will teach ourselves to use it. Essentially, it is possible to replace one behavior with another.

The same happens with our thoughts. The more often we repeat some thoughts, the more we teach ourselves to reproduce them unconsciously. If we change our thoughts consciously and repeat positive thoughts, then the negative will be replaced and if we insist they will stop.

6. Self adjustment- Self control

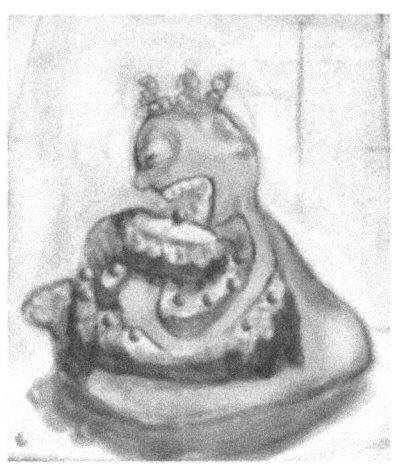

Self control is the ability we have to control ourselves to keep on or quit specific behaviors. In addition self control is the ability to overcome the internal desires and reactions and to control our behaviors. People who have a high self-control have better results in various fields such as social relationships, self management, and behaviors in their dietary control, keeping promises etc. Studies have shown that children with a high self-control grow more successful in all fields of their lives.

Low self-control is associated with a wide range of personal and interpersonal problems. People who have a low self-control appear to have an impulsive behavior such as control problems in eating, drinking alcohol and taking drugs. On the other hand, people who have extensively high levels of self-control produce pathological behaviors such as compulsions which are correlated with anxiety problems. If we want to change or to correct our self control, we should understand our behavior, define the specific changes and develop strategies to achieve the change. Self-regulation is based on self-observation, the awareness of situations and strategies that are used to achieve the change.

1st Stage: Self-observation

We draw conclusions from when we observe ourselves. We've already suggested an exercise for self-observation in which we observe the levels of hunger, the feelings of satisfaction, the emotions correlated with food and the emotions that provoke the consumption of food.

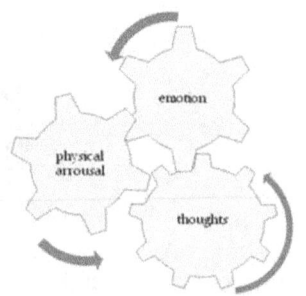

In the next step we need to understand that emotions cause thoughts, the thoughts feelings and how all that works for ourselves. We observe how the thoughts drive us to emotions, depending on each stimulus and how they are related to our emotions. To change our habits successfully, we should, first of all, understand their background in all fields, thoughts, behavior and emotions.

Let's ask ourselves the following:
- *What emotions do cause the stimulus for me to eat?*
- *What thoughts?*

- *Where do these thoughts lead me?*
- *Do my thoughts bring on emotions to me?*
- *Emotions bring me thoughts?*
- *Which are the physical symptoms caused by emotions?*
- *Which are the physical symptoms caused by thoughts?*
- *Do the physical symptoms worsen level of emotions?*
- *Do they change my behavior?*
- *Could I change my thoughts?*

CAUTION: in many cases our observation is selective and we refuse to admit some things. When the content and the accuracy of our self-observation are not objective, then the result will not be as successful as we want. A sincere conversation with close friends could lead us to valuable conclusions.

Examples (of the behavior) of overeating

Behavioral symptoms	Emotional symptoms
• Inability to stop or control eating • Fast consumption of large amounts of food • Eating even when we are not hungry • Secretly eating of large amounts and normal eating in front of others • Continuously eating during the day, not in specific meals	• Feeling of pressure which is relieved only by food consumption • Feeling of shame, frustration, sadness and remorse after eating large amounts of food • Lack of emotional satisfaction • Inability to control the feelings arising from our weight and our habits

2nd Stage: Self assessment

During the self-assessment stage, we need to understand and accept our problem. It is advisable to compare ourselves with others, even to accept comments from others to help us to see better the related behaviors. Sometimes there may be a refusal to accept certain behaviors.

The following questions could help us to understand our behavior:

- *Do I oversimplify or hyper analyze some situations?*
- *Am I absolutely sure about some issues?*
- *Do I make excuses even to myself?*
- *Do I generalize things and situations?*
- *Is my judgment based on my feelings?*
- *Do I ignore the positive aspects of myself?*

3rd Stage: Self-control

Self control is an ability which is fostered from our childhood. To be self controlled we should be able to regulate the rewards that are given to ourselves like to be patient when we are expecting something.

To display a behavior we are affected from our expectations for the results. We estimate the conflict between the possible choices, those with direct results and the results that need time to be come.

In the case of food intake, the short result is satisfaction and enjoyment of food and the long term result is weight loss if we are control it. People who have high self-control in their early behavior of eating and exercising take their reward in long term. They have better quality of life, better health, better body image etc. In contrast, those who have low self-control seek immediate satisfaction without having the patience to see the changes in their body.

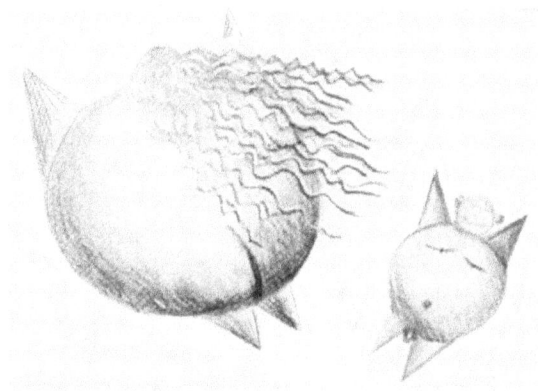

Also the common excuses like "I'll go on a diet from tomorrow" or "I will start a diet on Monday" give an extension to the behaviors of immediate satisfaction and extend the change of behaviors with a higher self control. In this way we find excuses for ourselves in order to continue our behavior as we are used to and avoid changes.

Of course, people with a high self-control sometimes fail to keep to the absolute program. But these people have cultivated the way of a corrective behavior. If they lose control when eating in a meal they will change their behavior by decreasing the food intake or by doing more exercise.

In contrast to people who have a low self-control don't change anything in their behavior in order to correct the mistakes. Instead they extend the date of expectant change of their behavior, but they never apply to their words. If we eat unhealthy foods then as long-term result it will be the worst quality of life, poorer health and worse body image. But we will have immediate gratification and pleasure. If we are patient and we recognize the positive changes in our bodies we will have better long term results.

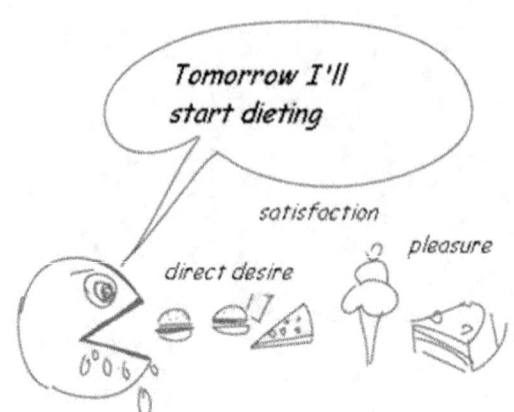

7.Nutrition

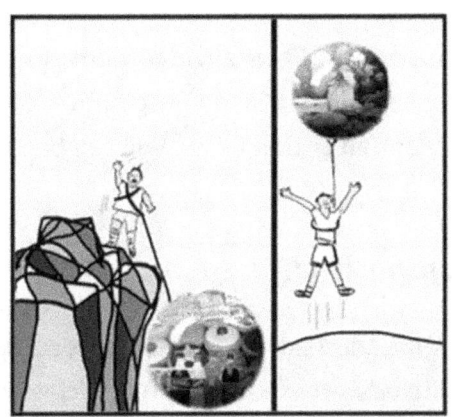

My body and the diet

To stay alive and be able to move, our body needs water and energy intake. The resting metabolic rate is the amount of energy that we need to stay alive without moving (breathing, heart function etc.). This amount is about 70% of the total energy we consume. In addition as many activities we have, the more energy we consume. The amount of energy in our body is measured by calories. 1 calorie is the energy required to raise the temperature of 1 gram of water for 1 degree of Celsius. 1000 calories are the famous kcal, usually used when we mention diets.

Body weight control

By eating we gain calories whereas by with exercising we burn calories. To maintain our body weight, the amount of energy we consume must be the same as the amount of energy we take. That means we burn and take the same amount of calories. When this is achieved we have a calorie balance.

The calories that we need to keep alive comprise our basic metabolism. The metabolic rate is influenced by a combination of factors such as the daily physical activity and nutrition as we will see bellow.

The body composition

Our body consists of fat and lean body mass that compose the total body weight. Lean mass includes the bones, the muscles, water and muscular tissue. Body fat consist visceral fat (liver, glands etc.) and fat storage. When somebody consumes more food than is needed then the adipose muscular tissue is increased and we get fatter.

The measurement of the percentage of body fat helps us to understand whether we have a normal body composition or not. To measure the percentage of fat in our body there are various methods. If the percentage is lower than the normal, that person is underweight, if it is above normal is the person obese. In men, the normal fat percentage ranges from 15% to 25% and in women from 18% to 35% in their total body weight.

Naturally women have more fat than men. Age increases the percentage normal limits of body fat in both sexes. The high percentage of body fat increases the risk for several diseases such as diabetes, hypertension and heart diseases. On the other hand, very low body fat disrupts the normal function in women.

Causes of malnutrition

Nutrition is the science that deals with food, nutrients in foods, actions, interactions and the balance of these in relation to health and diseases as well as the process by which the body breaks down, absorbs, transfers, uses and excretes nutrients in foods. Malnutrition could be caused by:

→ Excessive food intake
→ Poor quality of foods
→ Deficient diet

Let's ask ourselves...
- *Why do we eat some certain food when we know they are harmful?*

I know that with unhealthy foods...
- The extent of fat which is contained in snacks burden the liver.
- Light products may contain less fat but sometimes contain more sugar.
- The extra fat, extra salt and sugar make unhealthy food more delicious
- The intake of huge amount of fat prevents the brain to understand the feeling of satiety. So we become greedy.
- Experiments in animals have shown that snacks are addictive. Also sometimes maybe will developed withdrawal symptoms upon discontinuation of specific foods.

Food pyramid

The food pyramid has been developed using scientific data, in order to be used as a tool for healthy eating. It helps us to calculate the amount of each kind of nutrients we should contain in our diet.

On the top of the pyramid there are the foods that we should rarely eat, about once a week. At the bottom there are the foods that we should eat every day.

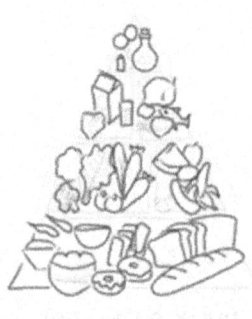

- The top of the pyramid contains fats, oils and sweets.
- In the second place there are foods that are rich in protein (meat, fish, poultry, legumes, eggs)
- In the third place there are the foods that contain vitamins (fruits and vegetables)
- At the base are the foods that are rich in carbohydrates (bread, rice, pasta, cereals, potatoes)

Let' ask ourselves...

- *Yesterday, did we eat foods that belong to each of the above categories?*
- *Are we used to eating foods from all the categories daily?*
- *How often do we eat food from each category?*
- *Do we compare the quantity that we should consume every day and the quantity we should consume weekly with what we eat?*

Nutrients

There are six main categories in which are classified the fifty nutrients that are necessary for the growth of our body:

Carbohydrates – are the main energy source for the body. There are simple and complex carbohydrates. Simple carbohydrates are found in sugar (glucose), in fruit (fructose). Complex carbohydrates are found in starchy foods such as pasta, bread, rice. Some foods are processed such as white rice and white flour while unprocessed foods such as whole grain bread are healthier because they contain more ingredients.

Fats – are essential for the main development of various hormones and they also protect the nervous system. Fats are divided into saturated and unsaturated. Saturated fats are present in all foods derived from animals such as milk, cheese and butter. Unsaturated fats are the fats derived from vegetables and are found in olive oil and nuts.

Proteins – are the building nutrition of the body. The proteins are the structural components of the cell. Cells by using proteins are reconstituted and replaced. Proteins are found in foods from vital origin such as meat, fish, eggs and milk. We must take one grammar of protein per each kilo of our weight each day. Children need about 1,5 grammar of protein per kilo because they are in their physical development.

Vitamins – cannot be created by our body and we receive them from food. They are needed in very small amounts for the growth and maintenance of a living organism. Vitamins are divided into water soluble (B, C, P) and fat soluble (A,D,E,K). Lack of vitamins can cause problems in our body. The sources of vitamins are fruits, vegetables, dairy, products wheat, nuts and legumes.

Metals and minerals - are inorganic elements that are necessary for our body in a minimum quantity. Metals and minerals are the macro elements (calcium, phosphorus, sulfur, potassium, sodium, chloride, magnesium) and trace elements (iron, fluorine, zinc. Copper, iodine, manganese, chromium and cobalt). They do not have any energy efficiency because that means they don't contain calories.

Water – the highest percentage of the human body and it is necessary to keep us alive. In our body water a solvent, lubricant, transport and is essential for thermoregulation of our body.

Exercise and diet

Those who exercise have a higher fuel requirement, which means more food. If we exercise systematically our body needs...

✓ More carbohydrates to have more endurance during exercise and better rehabilitation after exercise.
✓ More protein to build strong muscles
✓ More calcium to build strong bones
✓ More water to replace the fluids

We should eat 3-4 hours before healthy exercising, so that our body will have the time to digest the food. During exercise we should drink water frequently and if the exercise takes much time we need to take carbohydrates.

8. Exercise

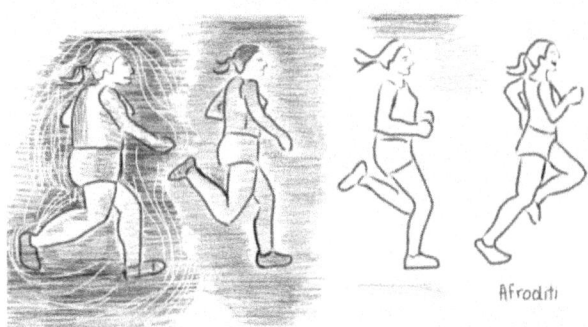

Afroditi

The benefits of exercise on our health

The exercise offers:
- ✓ More endurance, strength and muscle elasticity
- ✓ Greater resistance to diseases
- ✓ Weight control and obesity regulation
- ✓ Less fatigue and better performance in our daily lives
- ✓ Less musculoskeletal pain (mean, back and neck, joints)
- ✓ Prevention from heart problems
- ✓ Prevention from respiratory problems
- ✓ Reduces smoking, alcohol and other unhealthy habits
- ✓ Prevents the metabolic and neurological disorders
- ✓ Benefits effects of diseases such as hypertension, osteoporosis, diabetes and even cancer
- ✓ Better mood

- ✓ Less stress and tension
- ✓ Fun and pleasure
- ✓ Nice body and better appearance
- ✓ Greater self- confidence
- ✓ Better mental performance, concentration
- ✓ Better sleep
- ✓ Group and social relations, teamwork through exercise

> Surveys indicate that an underweighted person has a greater risk for health problems than somebody who is overweigh but doing exercise every day.
>
> The importance of exercise is very essential for our overall health

Benefits of exercise on mental health

Exercise increases energy and affects the mood of those who exercise regularly. Studies have shown that physical activity improves pour psychology:

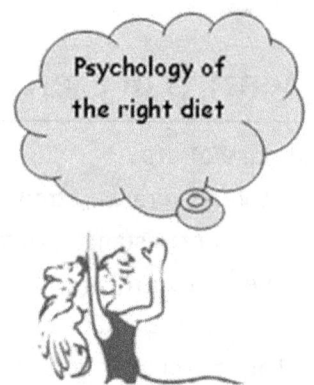

Psychology of the right diet

- ✓ Reduces the levels of anxiety and stress
- ✓ Improves mood disorders such as depression, anger and exhaustion
- ✓ Increases confidence
- ✓ Improves body image

Mainly, the changes in psychology are due to the preservation and enhancement of the physical health. In the neurophysiologic lever, exercise affects the substances which are produced in the body and affect the brain function. Also a good brain function depends directly on the blood flow which is affected by the cardiovascular diseases, sugar and reduced oxygenation of the brain cells.

> Exercise is the only natural way to develop and maintain the maximum oxygen intake, consequently increases oxygenation of the brain

Exercising improves the mental health and the well being. In addition to the physiological changes, exercise provides internal and external rewards. Exercising influences and shapes personality traits such as ethics, socialization and lifestyle. Any form of socializing boosts the mental health. Also, the personal improvement and the achievements of the goals are internal rewarding factors form of the person. These factors contribute in increasing the self-confidence and self-esteem.

Research on exercise and mental health

Exercising promotes the formation and the release of endogenous opioid which are endorphins and encephalins. Also, it increases the concentration levels of dopamine, norepinephrine and serotonin, neurotransmitters associated with our mood; it causes euphoria and softens the pain which is equivalent to the effect of antidepressants.

Compared to those who don't exercise, those who exercise have a greater self-esteem, better mood and they are more active. The body reacts better under stress conditions, releasing hormones in the blood such as cortisol and adrenaline. The antidepressant and anti-anxiety effects of exercise are confirmed. It seems that the most effective antidepressant treatment is a combination of exercise and antidepressants.

Exercise maintains high levels of cognitive functions which reduce aging, reduces the risk of dementia and Alzheimer. The risk of losing intellectual skills and memory is grater in people who don't exercise. The motor learning increases the number and the strength of synapses in the cerebellum.

Exercising contributes positively to sleep disorders. The duration of sleep and the measurements of EEG are higher in people who exercise. Positive effects have also shown in sleep the regulation of apnea syndrome.

Exercising for treating anxiety

A better result for stress reduction with exercise occurs when:
- ✓ The exercise is aerobic (running, swimming, cycling).
- ✓ The program is minimum 10-15 weeks long.
- ✓ Individuals have low fitness levels and high stress levels.
- ✓ The implementation of exercise combined with psychological therapy.

Exercise for treating depression

Exercise has better results in treating depression when:
- ✓ The endurance of the program is longer than 9 weeks.
- ✓ The exercise lasts long has a high intensity and is performed most of the days of the week.

Why don't I exercise?

To correct a behavior which does not satisfy us, we should analyze and understand it. Let's ask ourselves what is the reason we don't exercise.

Why don't I exercise?	Yes	No
I do not have free time to exercise because I will neglect the other jobs in my life		
I do not like to sweat		
My friends don't exercise, why should I?		
I don't like to exercise because I am not good at it		
It is so tiring to work out		
It is only for athletes		
I feel very well without exercise		
Exercise is a waste of time		
I do not find exercising enjoyable		
I do not want to push myself		

Metabolism

Our metabolism is defined as the rate at which our body burns calories when we are resting. The muscles are the organs that consume more energy. Big muscles consume more energy even when we are resting.

We know that for every 450 grammar of muscles our body needs about 14 calories a day. Every 450 grammars of adipose muscular tissue needs about 2 calories per day. So there is a huge difference between the burning energy in muscles and adipose muscular tissue.

People with developed muscles have a much better metabolism than those who are untrained. So to increase our metabolism we increase the muscle mass with the appropriate exercise. In this way, we improve the process of weight control.

> **Exercise builds our muscle mass and in this way we burn more calories**
> **Even when we are not exercising!**

Calorie consumption

Activity	calories
Walking	250
Gymnastics	310
Basketball	300
Swimming	320
Billiard	130
Bowling	208
Volleyball	350
Cycling	210
Football	540
Weight training	470
Rackets	600
Rope	700
Judo- karate	310
Running	650
Handball	600
Aerobic dance	420
Dance	264

With the physical activity we consume 15-30% of our daily total energy. People who exercise daily consume much more energy than people who don't work. Physical activity is more effective for the treatment of obesity and to control the rate of fat when people exercise for a longer period of time. In the table are presented the calories we burn every hour in different activities.

Put physical activity in my life

Before we start exercising we should make some medical examinations. We slowly begin working out in a low intensity and gradually increase duration and intensity. Excessive exercise, especially when we started it could lead to exhaustion and injuries.

We find the kind of exercise that best fits to our lifestyle and our character, whether it is going to the gym, dancing, cycling, swimming, hiking, team sports etc. If we like what we do, then we get more satisfaction and the chances of working out regularly are increased.

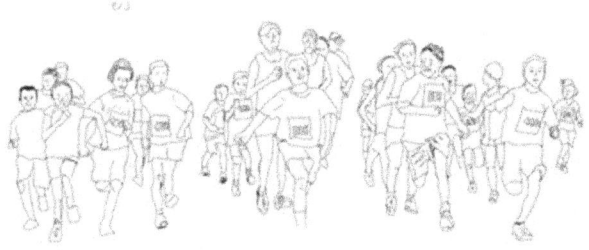

Types of exercise

Physical activity can be divided into two categories aerobic and anaerobic exercise.

Aerobic exercise involves the movement of large muscle masses during a continuous period. We work large muscle groups for a long duration and low intensity. Aerobic exercise involves the following activities:

✓ Running	✓ Swimming	✓ Aerobic
✓ Fast walking	✓ Cycling	✓ Dancing

When we include aerobic exercise as a part of our daily routine, the heart and the cardiovascular system will be improved. Furthermore, our mood is improved because exercise releases stress and anxiety. **Anaerobic exercise** builds strong muscles and includes activities such as:

- Weight training
- Resistance machines
- Exercises with body weight
- Isometric exercises e.g. yoga -pilates

Only 20 minutes of aerobic exercise a day can cause significant changes in the shape of our body and our overall physical condition. The development of muscle mass helps to protect bones that are extremely important for everyone.

The sport games are a combination of aerobic and anaerobic exercise. They've performed continuously, with very short breaks and contain phases with strong efforts. The sport games are a very nice way to exercise while playing a game. The body and the mind revitalize while at the same time we have fun.

Record my daily workout

The daily monitoring of workout is an important way of reward, because we see it all written down. In the following table we can list the time and the type of physical activity for one week.

Calendar of physical activity		
	Physical activity description	Duration
Monday		
Tuesday		
Wednesday		
Thursday		
Friday		
Saturday		
Sunday		

I make the curve of my monthly physical activity

In the horizontal column the days of the month listed and in the vertical column the time of our daily work out. The resulting curve will show us the image of all the month. The schematic illustration of our workout will tone our confidence and motivate us for more effort. Also, at a glance we could compare months and see our improvement.

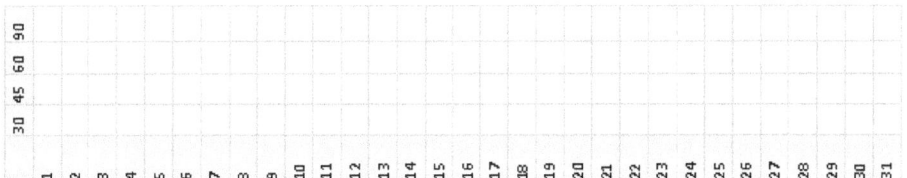

9. Changing eating and exercise habits

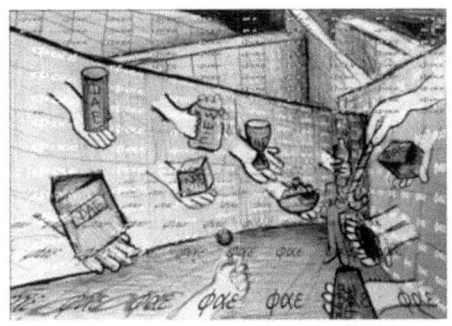

As we saw, if we want to change our behavior we first of all should understand it. The observation of our behaviors and the analysis of our thoughts and feeling is the most important step. The golden rule is to be honest with ourselves in order to carry on the right way.

In the stage of self-evaluation, we identify the points that we should intervene. The changes will be very small and will adopt permanently. Those changes will not deprive us and we will be satisfied with ourselves. Then if we are satisfied by ourselves more small changes will follow more easily, until we have the final result.

The essence is to change our lifestyle in a positive way without oppression. To do this we should reward all small efforts for change and avoid small mistakes. Even a change one or two times per week is important to the final result.

We try to have a clear opinion of every behavior. For that reason we analyze separately the behavior of nutrition to the behavior of exercise. We should not relate the changes that we make in each field. This is a common error that people do when dealing the problems in their lives. Each theme has its own special place in our lives. If somebody confuses all the different categories then he could easily lose control and give up. That's why we should try to separate them.

Suggestions to change and enhance eating behaviors

We try to:

- ✓ Eat only at predetermined hours
- ✓ Eat only at predetermined places
- ✓ Not combine eating with other activities
- ✓ Not go to places with temptations- like fast foods, patisseries etc
- ✓ Buy foods only if after we've eaten
- ✓ Place the foods in specific places
- ✓ Take the required nutrients
- ✓ Eat foods that contain calcium
- ✓ Reduce sugar intake
- ✓ Eat enough fiber
- ✓ Gradually reduce the calorie intake
- ✓ Moderate salt intake
- ✓ Moderate fat intake
- ✓ Increase fluid intake
- ✓ Minimize alcohol intake

We substitute unhealthy habits with healthy choices

Unhealthy	Healthy
White bread	Whole wheat bread or multigrain
Cereals with chocolate	Whole grains
Fried potatoes or fried vegetables	Roasted potatoes, boiled vegetables, or raw
Sweets and foods with a lot of sugar	Fruits
Milk, yogurt and cheese with high fat	Milk, yogurt and cheese with low fat
Meats	Fish, poultry, eggs, chops
Mayonnaise, butter, margarine	Olive oil, fish oil, vegetable oil
Cheese pie	Bun
Soft drinks	Juice
Fried foods	Grilled foods

When we go out we can order healthy foods:
- ✓ We prefer grilled meat or fish
- ✓ We prefer baked potatoes than fried
- ✓ We order salads without many sauces but olive oil
- ✓ We order pizza with vegetables and not a lot of sausages
- ✓ We request black bread
- ✓ We avoid soft drinks

From the table of last chapter we note the unhealthy habits and we change them with healthy ones.

Unhealthy habits	Replace with healthy

We change our thoughts:

→ Change our expectations on what is delicious and what is not. Tasty foods are healthy foods.
→ People who eat healthy foods have more attractive body because it is more healthy
→ We think mentally how our body and our health will be in the future if we eat in a healthy way
→ We write down a list of what we ate every day
→ We talk about what's on the list with close friends and family

---

The best way to lose weight and maintain a stable weight is to adopt permanently healthy eating habits

---

We adopt healthy habits

The slight calorie increase leads to gradual weight loss.
✓ We frequently participate in physical activities
✓ We play sports and not on the pc
✓ We get sufficient rest
✓ We reduce sedentary habits like watching TV
✓ The choose to go out for a walk with friends
✓ We use stairs and walking when we are on the move
✓ We learn new sports
✓ We use the bike for our transportation

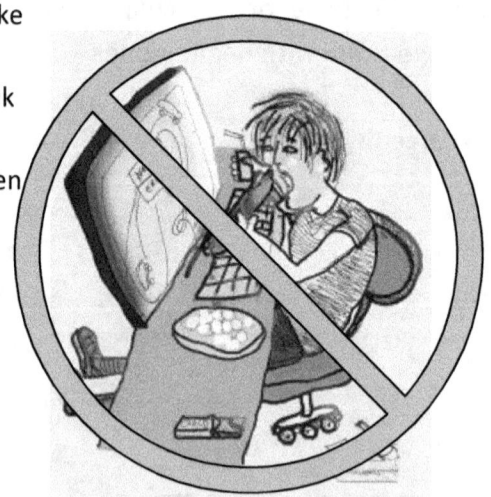

10.   Goals in diet

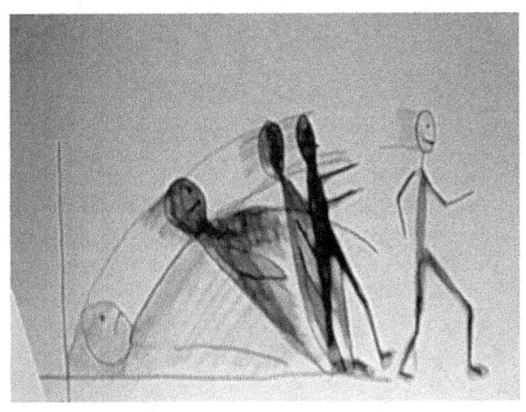

We should set goals in everything we want to achieve in our lives. In weight management we have to set goals related with the behaviors of exercise and nutrition. If we set right goals, the result of change will be achieved more easily and effectively. The right goals will guide us step by step to change related habits with eating routines and physical activity.

When we complete our goals unconsciously and consciously we reward ourselves. Thus we develop internal awards that enhance our behavior while we increase our self-confidence and our self-esteem. After the completion of the goals we move to the next one with a better attitude and faith that we'll succeed.

Rules of setting goals

When we follow the rules of setting goals then the chances of success are higher.

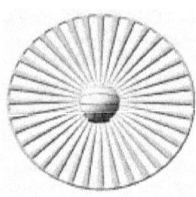

Specific

The goals "I will get slim" or "from Monday I will make diet" are general. We should define our behavior as much as possible. So these objectives should be specific:
Examples:
I will lose a pound next month, I will adhere to the diet program, I will replace my fried food with grilled and boiled.
I will walk a half an hour every day, I will walk 4 times a week.

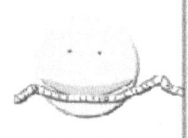

Measurable

Measurable goals are showing exactly the effort that we have to do in order to achieve. For example, eat only a sweet during the week is a goal that controls the amount of sweets. For the exercise we can set as a goal to go to the gym for 1 hour 3 times per week.
Examples:
Exercising 1 hour 3 times per week.
Specific amounts of food, specific meals by following a program

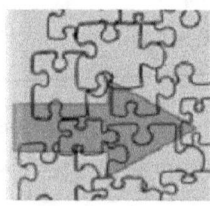

Short term goals

Short term goals are related to near future. To achieve a long term goal we need a lot of time. For example to lose 5 pounds we have to break it down to smaller pieces.
In this way we define the process and the steps that we have to achieve. In this way, we can control much better a long term goal. The goal is controlled better and doesn't seem frustrating.

The same happens with for the exercising. If we want to exercise an hour every day we should gradually start with 45 minutes 3 times a week and add a little more each week according to our abilities.
Examples:
The goal to loose 5 kg, can be divided into 2 segments. 2,5 kg per month or 1 kg every 2 weeks is heard easier to be achieved.
The same happens with exercising, if we want to exercise an hour every day we will begin working out 20-30 min and gradually increase the intensity and duration.

The following table identifies the type of goals. We should try to meet these requirements for our goals. In this way we check whether the goals are correctly determined.

Personal goals for dieting & exercising up until the following week	Question I'm obliged to answer Is my goal...?			
	Specific	Long-term	Measured	Realistic and controlled
To start a diet	-	-	-	-
To start exercising	-	-	-	-
To lose a kilo	✓	-	✓	✓
To keep to my diet program	✓	✓	✓	✓
To walk for 30 minutes 4 time a week	✓	✓	✓	✓

Goals monitoring

The success of the goals is also depends on the monitoring. We should check the progress of our goals and modify them if it is necessary. If a goal is not held we need to repeat or change it before moving on this way, we don't stray from our long term goal.

To properly monitor our goals is better to record them. We can use a table in which we will define our long term goal and then split it to short term goals per month. If it is necessary, we change short term goals after checking their progress.

In the following table we record our daily goals. The recording of daily goals maybe performed every week or every two weeks. We indicate the annual and monthly goal to understand better the smaller short term goals. Then we can copy these data to the annual table. The record of successful efforts motivates us and gives us a lot of confidence.

GOALS OF THE YEAR:			
SIX MONTHS GOALS	DATE	CHANGES	FOLLOW UP
MONTHLY GOAL			
WEEKLY GOAL			
DAILY GOAL	DATE	CHANGES	FOLLOW UP
MONDAY			
TUESDAY			
WEDNESDAY			
THURSDAY			
FRIDAY			
SATURDAY			
SUNDAY			

Team goals

The power of a team is greater than the power of each person separately. There is the strength of commitment to the group and the support of each person separately. For this reason, when we set the team goals we are more effective.

Team goals should be recorded and posted in conspicuous places that will be accessible for all the members of the group. The headline of the team's goals could be the message of the group. This message should spur all the members in a collective effort to adopt the behavior which expresses the team.

11. Change of the behavior

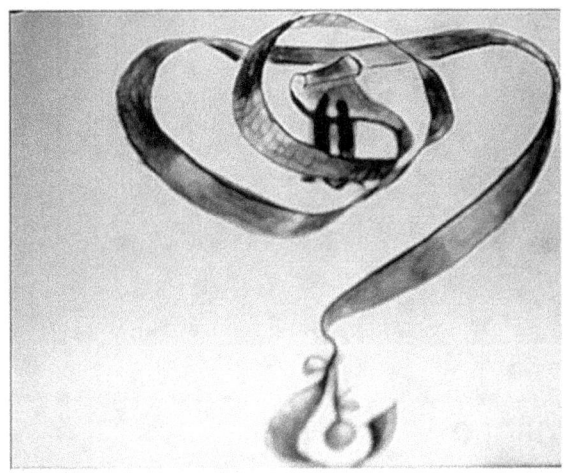

To change our behavior successfully, we should know where to intervene. In the below picture, the behavior is influenced by several factors. Of course we cannot change factors such as genes and the environment where we have grown up. We know that we can change our thinking and our way of life, that is something that will also affect our feelings.

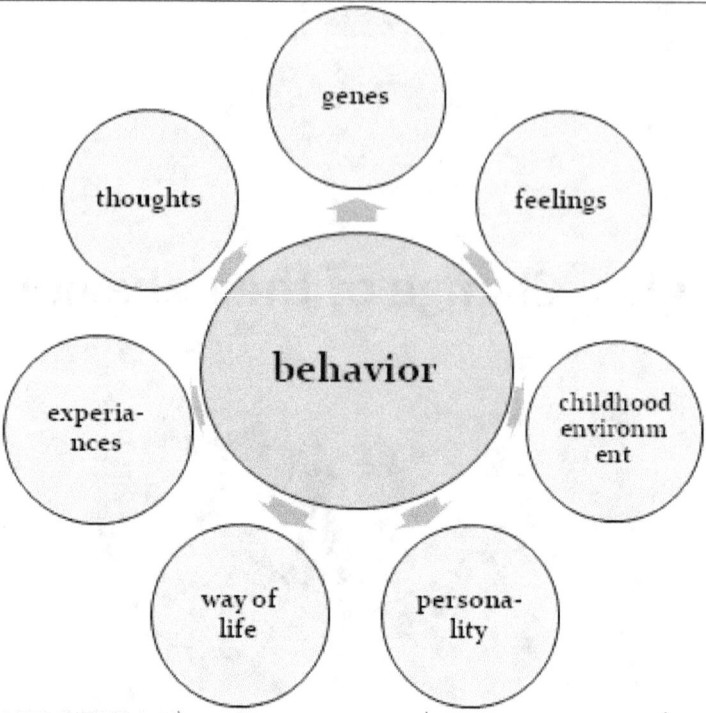

Stages of change

To change our unhealthy behaviors and adopt healthy ones we should be determined and confident that we can change them. Understanding the stages of change helps us to understand why, when and how it is possible to change. The stages of change are:

1. I have not thought so far that I should watch my diet
2. I am thinking about changing my diet next month
3. The Last month I made some attempts to change my diet
4. Last month I watched my diet very much
5. The last six months I watch my diet very much

Let's think...

- *At what stage am I?*
- *What do I have to do to change my stage?*

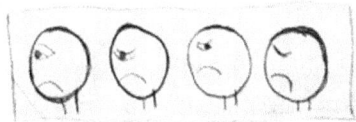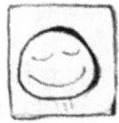

After we observe in which stage we are, we state the stages to move forward. We are maybe at a stage and progress to the next or reverse to the previous. In order the change to be effective we should be determined that we can do that, so we are in a phase of action. By understanding the stage that we are in, contributes to the success of our efforts.

To get active we must be determined that we can do it. During the preparation phase we plan to change and identify what we want to change. At the same time we define the time that we start changing. The following questions will help us start. We must not forget that our goal is to change the way we live.

- *What do I want to change and what do I accept for myself?*
- *To what extent can I change?*
- *Can I rely on myself to change?*
- *What are my goals?*
- *What is my motivation?*
- *How strong are my motives?*
- *What will my effort be?*
- *Is it worth the effort?*
- *How do I see myself in the future?*

The theory of change is a cognitive process. Cognitive processes increase knowledge, awareness and understanding of the benefits. They are related to the understanding of ourselves and the change of our thoughts and behaviors. Self-awareness helps us to make the start. The understanding and the acceptance of a problem is the trigger for the solution.

To begin the change:
1. We recognize the problem
2. We observe and record our behavior
3. We define the parts where we have to interfere
4. We set ways for behavioral changes
5. We find alternative behaviors

Which are the changes that we should make?

We all know what our mistakes are when we don't lose weight. If we identify and record those mistakes then the possibilities to change are even more effective. If we observe the table in the 2nd chapter we will find were we should intervene. The following questions could be helpful: Where should I make the changes in my behavior?

- *At the time of meals*
- *In the amount of food*
- *In the quality of food*
- *In the connections between food and emotions*
- *In the bad habits*

> Repeat: The best way to lose and maintain our weight is to adopt permanently healthy eating and exercise habits. And change the way of life

Motivation

Before we make the effort to change our behavior, we need to calculate the motivation that will lead us to a positive result. If we don't have an important motivation then the successful changes are decreased.

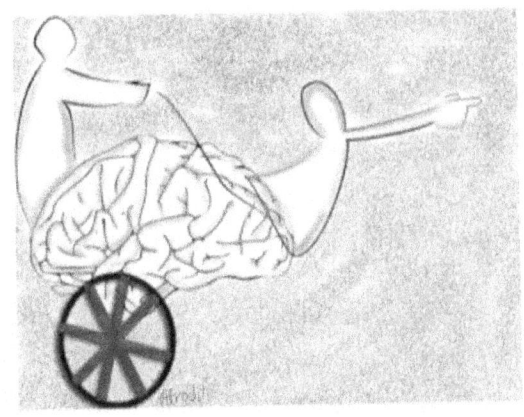

The motivation is divided into internal and external. Internal motives are those which cover our own expectation and external are those that meet the expectations of our environment. To determine the significance of our internal motivation we should answer the following questions:

- *Why is it important to me?*
- *Do I have the correct expectations?*
- *Am I pressured by others to change myself?*

The change of behavior should start from the person himself because of his determination and not be the result of external pressure. Besides, every person is responsible for the modification of their behavior.

Strengthening of our behavior

To strengthen our behavior there are several ways:

- **Positive self-reward.** We use positive self reward to reinforce ourselves for the effort we make. Frequent rewards may sound excessive sometimes. But the rewards significantly increase our internal motivation. Generally those who have a high self confidence reward themselves more often than those who have a low self-confidence.

- **Negative self-reward.** A negative self reward is more often used than a positive. We are often disappointed by ourselves and we use negative thoughts to motivate us. Some people prefer the negative self-reward than the positive. However, the positive award is much more effective than the negative.

- **Rewards.** If rewards are used properly it could be an important motivation for our behavior. The rewards in a diet program should never be associated with foods or sweets. It is a general mistake to reward ourselves with a big treat, just because we reduce food intake. Instead, we should reward ourselves every time we successfully complete a reduced meal. The reward could be a trip, a present, etc.

- **Self-punishment.** Many times we make the mistake and we consider the whole process of dieting as a self-punishment. The diet should be implemented as a process of permanent change of our behavior on diet and 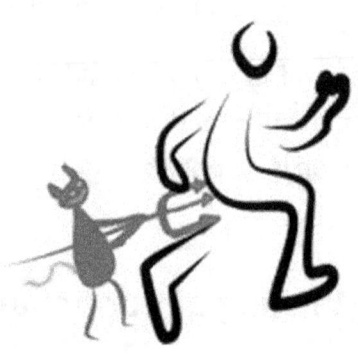 exercise and not something we are forced to do.

- **Positive thoughts.** Positive thoughts drive us to positive attitudes and repetition of desired behaviors. If we have negative attitudes towards a behavior then it is more likely it isn't continued. Also positive thoughts boost our confidence and develop positive feelings for the desired behavior. Even more, positive thoughts help to reduce symptoms of anxiety and depression.

Modify our expectations

To change our behavior radically we must change the way we think. In the 4th chapter we learnt how to observe and analyze our thoughts. Also it is very important to understand that our thoughts are associated with our emotions and what are the changes are taking place in our behavior.

In theory everything seems easy, but in practice things are a little more difficult. In the beginning we should consciously try to change the way we think. According to the behavioral theory, when we consciously repeat a behavior or some thoughts, we adopt them after several repetitions.

The expectations are also a key to the required result. Our expectations are relevant to the reward we get from our behavior and simultaneously provide a strong motivation for the repetition of the desired behavior.

To adopt a behavior permanently we must have positive expectations from it. To lose weight is a positive expectation but the result of the effort will take time. Each behavior should be rewarded immediately. Related with diet we can adopt the following expectation:

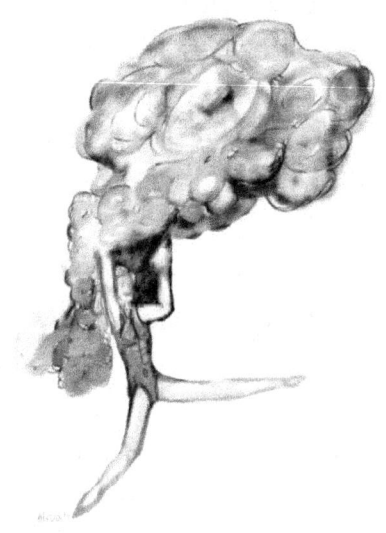

✓ **Tasty foods are healthy foods**
When we eat something healthy, we

should try to feel the benefits in our body. The opposite should happen when we eat something that is unhealthy. We try to feel the differences in our body when we eat healthy and when we eat unhealthy foods.

✓ **Exercise directly benefits our health**

It is the same with the nutrition. We should try to feel the benefits in our body immediately after the exercise, also during the exercise. We shouldn't wait to get slim to recognize the value of exercise. We always try to a positive feedback from what is happening in our body.

✓ **We show ourselves healthy standards**

People who eat healthy and exercise daily have leaner bodies and are healthier.

We reward our effort

Even if we break the rules we should always use nice words when we think of ourselves. Continuously belittling ourselves leads to decreased self-esteem and self-confidence. We must always try to maintain high self confidence and self-esteem. So instead of feeling guilty when we eat something unhealthy, we reward ourselves when we eat something healthy.

We should not be hard with ourselves, instead of focusing on the fact that we do not like healthy food, it is better to focus on the positive expectations and positive results. We strongly reward ourselves when we exercise. We announce our success to those close to us and must receive a reward. It is wrong to belittle ourselves. It is also a big mistake to allow others to belittle us too. We should search for strength and not the negative judgment.

12. Psychological techniques

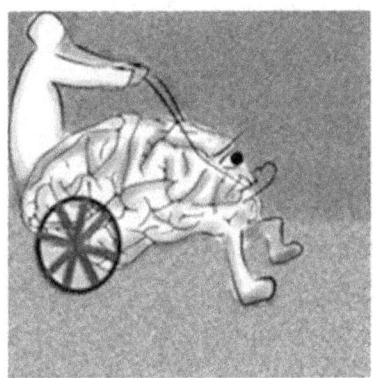

Imagery: we imagine ourselves in the future

Imagery is the fantastic representation of ourselves or fantastic situations. We could imagine everything, behaviors, thoughts, feelings, movements etc. It has been shown that the method of visualization uses neuro-cognitive mechanisms and could cause changes in our brain and in our way of thinking.

Studies have shown that when we want to make a change first of all we should accept it. When we get slimmer, our body image changes. When we lose 5 or 10 kilos, our body image does not change dramatically. But when we lose many pounds the image of our body changes a lot.

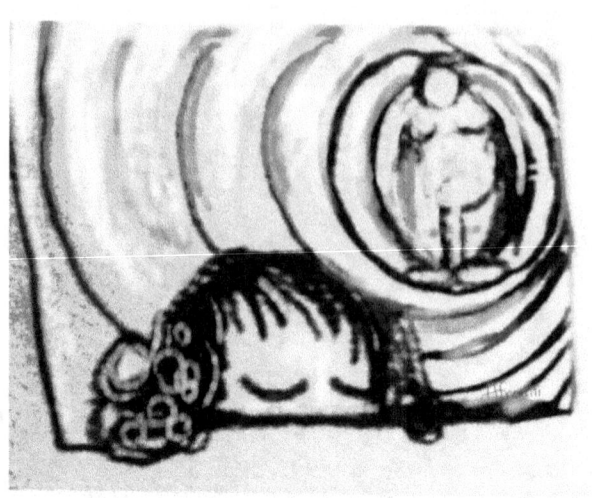

The change of the image often limits the final result, for people who lose a lot of weight. Sometimes people refuse to change the image of their body. Many behaviors are hidden behind that image. That psychological barrier could be overcome only if we get in terms with the change. The best way to accept that change is to use imagery. Imagery is used widely by athletes to change the associated behaviors with their performance. It has been found that by imagery practicing brain synapses change.

In order the imagery on diet to have positive result we should:
- ✓ Imagine that we can effectively control our behavior
- ✓ Imagine that we have a new slimmer body which we enjoy
- ✓ We feel pleasure from our new look
- ✓ We imagine that we are trying new clothes
- ✓ We imagine that we use our body, we dance, swim, run, flirt etc.
- ✓ Imagine that people in our environment accept us more than before
- ✓ Imagine that we have to overcome some problems

Self talk

Self talk is the dialogue that we do with ourselves. It is our inner "little voice" that tell us what to do. We all use self-talk, sometimes more and sometimes less. Basically self talk expresses the thoughts for ourselves and the behaviors that we are planning to do.

Most of the times, this "little voice" condemns us and thinks negatively. People who have high confidence use more positive self-talk. To change our thoughts successfully we can consciously change our self-talk. Thus we influence our thoughts like our behavior.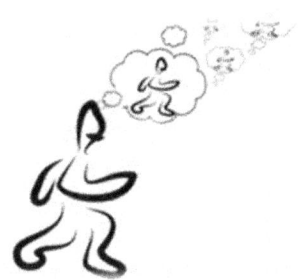

Development of self-confidence

Certainly the person who believes in himself will accomplish much more than somebody else who has doubts about his abilities. The faith in ourselves means faith in a successful effort. The development of self-confidence is very important for the success in all areas of life.

It is much easier to focus on the negative characteristics of our self as we do with negative thoughts. People who criticize themselves argue that they do it because they are objective and judge themselves without excesses. But if we don't recognize the positive aspects of our character we will have a low self-esteem.

We should give importance to our success as small as they are. Dealing with failure is a key that everybody should learn from an early age. In cases of failure we should focus on what we have to correct it rather than face the frustration and criticizing.

To increase our confidence:

✓ We make a list of our success no matter how small they are
✓ We don't think about failure in our future actions
✓ We define goals that satisfy us not others
✓ We learn to face failure and learn from our mistakes
✓ We don't allow to feel rejected
✓ We imagine a successful profile in the future
✓ We learn relaxation techniques and stress management

Relaxation techniques

Relaxation techniques are commonly used to treat anxiety and stress. In general, those techniques are very effective. People who apply relaxation techniques in their daily lives are calmer and they have better self-control. As we saw, food intake is associated with the relief of intense feelings such as anxiety. Relaxation techniques could replace that connection. That means when we are in great tension, instead of relieving that emotion with food we calm down with those techniques.

The following are some forms of relaxation techniques:

Breathing techniques, when we breathe calmly it is also quite slow and deep. On the other hand, when we are tense, our breath is fast and sharp. When we change consciously our breath, we have very good results in relaxation. We have to concentrate on our breathing characteristics such as the diaphragm, the chest, the duration of inhale and exhale. The simplest method of breathing relaxation proposes to inhale for 4 seconds and exhale for 6 seconds. This duration may vary depending on lung capacity and our physical condition. That exercise could be carried out for 1 minute, 2 minutes or 10 to 20 repetitions. Each one could develop a program of breathing that fits to him. With constant practice and experience the relaxation is faster and more efficient.

Autogenic training, performed by focusing attention on physical observations in our body. The focus could be given to the weight, the heat, the pulses, breath and specific parts of the body.

Biofeedback technique, performed by observing the symptoms of anxiety. The observation of all the physical symptoms of stress could help in controlling them.

Progressive muscle relaxation. With this technique we practice the tension and relaxation of our muscles. In this way we feel the difference between tension and relaxation and try to understand it. After that recognition we should try to eliminate tension when we notice it.

The commitment

The environment affects each person's intentions to change our behavior. The commitment to significant people is proved effective to the final goal. These people could help us to:

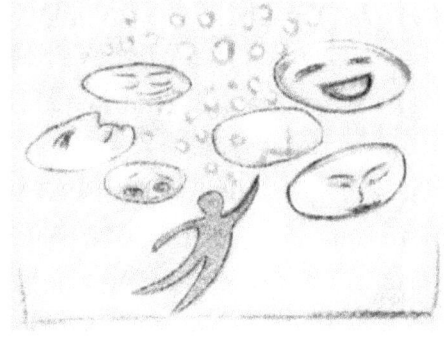

- ✓ **Push us in starting a new effort**
- ✓ **Help us during the effort**
- ✓ **Support us psychologically**

Also it is very effective when we start an effort with people who have common goals. In those cases we share the difficulties, the pain and reward each other.

Planning

We know that if we pass long periods without eating anything then our body needs to fill the gap and usually ends up with overeating. A diet plan regulates our biorhythms. Thus our body learns to balance and effectively we could control overeating.

As we have seen, our goal when is to want to lose weight we should follow a diet and an exercise program without pressing ourselves to eat less or to avoid a meal. The most effective way is to prepare our planning at the beginning of the week or month. After a while the program will become a habit. People who control their weight properly have small frequent meals. With a little effort we can achieve that by regulating our daily habits.

The weekly diet program helps us to prepare also a shopping list that we need and not stray in our shopping. It has been observed that when we don't know what we want to shop we easily buy unhealthy foods. The detailed planning will help us even more. If we monitor our diet program, it is very important. Proper monitoring will help us to make the appropriate changes where necessary.

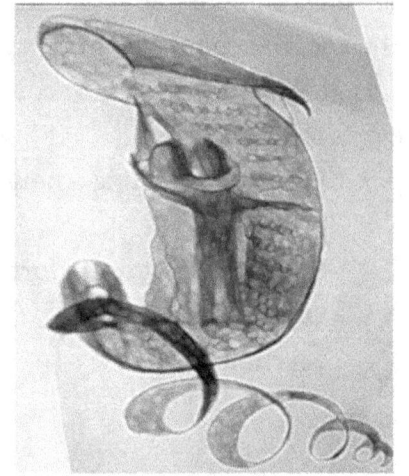

Time	Quantity	Monitoring

Overcoming the impediments

A proper definition of goals means the programming of exercise and diet behaviors. The rule for realistic goals helps us to prevent irregularity because we don't ask from ourselves to do something absurd. We check our goals and always have our behavior under observation and use these valuable conclusions to improve ourselves.

We create the appropriate situations not only in our psychology, but also in our environment, trying to anticipate situations but also reduce temptations. For this reason we won't buy foods such as sweets or snacks that can be consumed while being in an emotional release. It is better not to have these foods at home if we cannot control the consumption.

Prevention is the best way to control our behavior. By predicting the obstacles that may arise it is better to give solutions in the effort to control our weight. It will be perfect if we could predict the situation and not let it create problems at all. Also we observe if a problem is real or it is an excuse to avoid specific behaviors. In the following table we identify the obstacles and we propose solutions overcome them.

- ✓ we set our goals
- ✓ prevent problems
- ✓ use conclusions
- ✓ form right situations
- ✓ reduce external stimulus
- ✓ usage of control techniques

Possible obstacles	Possible solutions
The canteen at work has not healthy foods	1. I take healthy foods from home 2. We ask to increase variety of healthy foods 3. I do not eat anything
Fast food meals are unhealthy	I get healthy foods from home
I don't have time to exercise	Probably it is an excuse. Everybody could find half an hour 3 times a week.

Tips

➔ We study the table in the previous section where we recorded the weekly physical activity. What we should do to improve our health and our weight? We must modify the type and the amount of the time we spent per week in physical activity as follows:

- ✓ In the frequency..........................
- ✓ In the duration.............................
- ✓ In the type of exercise.................

→ We create by ourselves a balanced diet according to the following rules:

- 3 main meals (breakfast, lunch, dinner) in the proportion of nutrients that should be consumed daily (50-60% carbohydrates, 30% fats and 15% proteins at every meal).
- We add 2 more light meals between the basics meals (brunch, afternoon) which may include fruits, nuts, dairy products etc.
- Our weekly diet should includes all types of food

→ We make a healthy recipe book. Everyone in the family can propose favorite healthy recipes. We can write and also take pictures. The healthy book for the family.

References

- Andrade, A. M., Coutinho, S. R., Silva, M. N., Mata, J., Vieira, P. N., Minderico, C. S., και συν. (2010). The effect of physical activity on weight loss is mediated by eating self-regulation. *Patient Education and Counseling 79* , σσ. 320–326.
- Baker, R., & Kirschenbaum, D. (1993). Self-monitoring may be necessary for successful weight control. *Behavioral Therapy, 24* , σσ. 377-394.
- Ball, K., Crawford, D., & Kenardy, J. (2004). Longitudinal Relationships among Overweight, Life Satisfaction, and Aspirations in Young Women. *Obesity Research , 12* (6), σσ. 1019-1030.
- Bartholomew, K. L., Parcel, G. S., Kok, G., & Gottlieb, N. H. (2006). *Planning Health Promotion Programs: An Intervention Mapping Approach.* San Francisco: Jossey-Bass.
- Baueister, R. F., Heatherton, T. F., & Tice, D. M. (1994). *Losing Control: How and Why People Fail at Self-Regulati.* San Diego: Academic Press.
- Bodenheimer, T., & Handley, M. (2009). Goal-setting for behavior change in primary care: An exploration and status report. *Patient Education and Counseling 76* , σσ. 174-180.
- Boekaerts, M., Zeidner, M., & Pintrich, P. R. (2000). *Handbook of Self-Regulation.* San Diego, California: Elsevier Academic Press.
- Brennan, L., Walkley, J., Fraser, S. F., Greenway, K., & Wilks, R. (2008). Motivational interviewing and cognitive behaviour therapy in the treatment of adolescent overweight and obesity: Study design and methodology. *Contemporary Clinical Trials 29* , σσ. 359–375.
- Cash, T. &. (2002). *Body image: A handbook of theory, research, and clinical practice.* New York: Guilford Press.
- Foster, G. D., Makris, A. P., & Bailer, B. A. (2005). Behavioral treatment of obesity. *American Journal of Clinical Nutrition, 82* , σσ. 230S–5S.
- Gottfredson, M. R. (2011). *Self-Control Theory.* Ανάκτηση January 06, 2011, από Blackwell Encyclopedia of Sociology:
- Korkeila, K. M., Rissanen, A., Koskenvuo, M., & Sorensen, T. (1998). Predictors of Major Weight Gain in Adult Finns: Stress, Life Satisfaction and Personality Traits. *International Journal of Obesity , 22* (10), σσ. 949-957.
- Malterud, K., & Ulriksen, K. (2010). "Norwegians fear fatness more than anything else"—A qualitative study of normative newspaper messages on obesity and health. *Patient Education and Counseling, 81* , σσ. 47-52.
- Ratzan, S. C. (2004). Sllent threat: Non-communicable disease and obesity. *Journal of Health Communication 9* , σσ. 1-2.

• Roberts, R. E., Strawbridge, W. J., Deleger, S., & Kaplan, G. A. (2002). Are the Fat More Jolly? *Annals of Behavioral Medicine , 24* (3), σσ. 169-180.

• Schmeichel, B. J., Harmon-Jones, C., & Harmon-Jones, E. (2010). Exercising Self-Control Increases Approach Motivation. *Journal of Personality and Social Psychology , 99* (1), σσ. 162-173.

• Θεοδωράκης, Γ., & Χασάνδρα, Μ. (2006). Σχεδιασμός προγραμμάτων Αγωγής Υγείας. Εκδ. Χριστοδουλίδη. Θεσσαλονίκη.

• Θεοδωράκης, Γ., Παπαϊωάννου Α. (2002). Το προφίλ μαθητών με βάση υγιεινές και ανθυγιεινές συμπεριφορές: Σχέσεις με τον αθλητισμό. *Ψυχολογία, 9,* 547-562.

• Θεοδωράκης, Ι. (1990). Άσκηση και Υγεία: Πως η φυσική αγωγή θα μας πείσει για ένα δια βίου αθλητικό τρόπο ζωής. *Αθλητική Ψυχολογία ,* σσ. 37-54.

• Καλπάκογλου, Θ. (2001). Γνωσιακή-συμπεριφοριστική θεραπεία. Στο Π. Ασημάκης, *Σύγχρονες ψυχοθεραπείες απο τη θεωρία στην εφαρμογή* (σσ. 284-324). Αθήνα: Ασημάκης.

• Παπαϊωάννου, Αθ., Θεοδωράκης, Γ., & Γούδας, Μ. (2003). *Για μια καλύτερη φυσική αγωγή.* Θεσσαλονίκη: Χριστοδουλίδη.

• Σίμος, Γ. (2010). Η γνωστική συμπεριφορική θεραπεία της παχυσαρκίας. *Εγκέφαλος, 47 (2)* .

Internet References:
http://hellas.teipir.gr/Thesis/Trofima/pinakes/galaktomika/galaktomika_open.htm
www.medlook.net
http://www.hsph.harvard.edu/nutritionsource/what-should-you-eat/pyramid/
World Health Organization: http://www.who.int/nutrition/en/
BBC health treatments:
http://www.bbc.co.uk/health/treatments/healthy_living/nutrition/

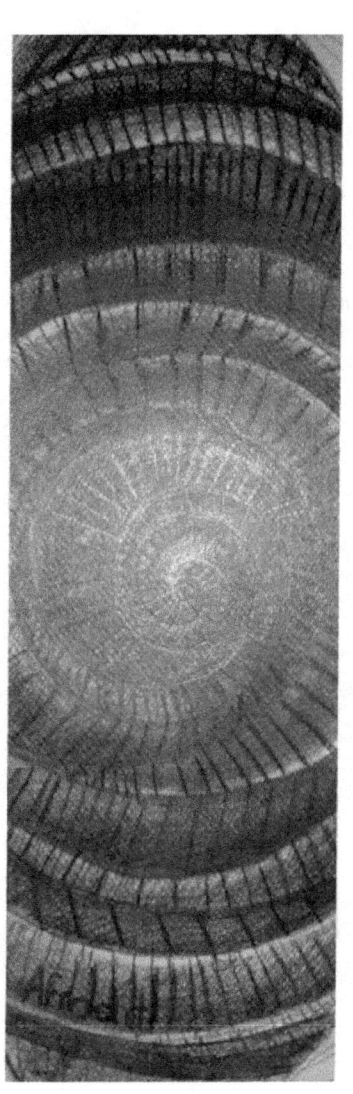

CV

Lina Psouni born in 1978 in Chania Greece. She has the first BSc in Physical education and sport science and the second in Psychology. Also she has MSc in maximizing athletic performance with thesis subject in Sport Psychology. Now she is a doctoral candidate at the University of Thessaly.

In parallel with studies she was a water polo athlete. She won the world champion with the juniors' women water polo national team of Greece and the champion of Greece. Now she is doing a lot of sports like beach volley, sailing and triathlon.

Her scientific interests are in the areas of health psychology, weight management, sports psychology, attitude and behavior relationships. She has published in Greek and foreign conferences and writes articles in the press and the internet. At the same time she makes seminars in sports psychology and health psychology.